Managing the "Drugs" in Your Life

Managing the "Drugs" in Your Life

A PERSONAL AND FAMILY GUIDE TO THE RESPONSIBLE USE OF DRUGS, ALCOHOL, MEDICINE

STEPHEN J. LEVY, Ph.D.

McGRAW-HILL BOOK COMPANY

New York   St. Louis   San Francisco   Auckland   Bogotá   Guatemala
Hamburg   Johannesburg   Lisbon   London   Madrid   Mexico
Montreal   New Delhi   Panama   Paris   San Juan   São Paulo
Singapore   Sydney   Tokyo   Toronto

1 2 3 4 5 6 7 8 9 DOC DOC 8 7 6 5 4

ISBN 0-07-037411-2{H.C.}
      0-07-037448-1{PBK.}

First Paperback Edition, 1984

LIBRARY OF CONGRESS CATALOGING IN PUBLICATION DATA

Levy, Stephen J.
Managing the drugs in your life.
1. Drugs—Popular works.   2. Medication abuse.
3. Drug abuse.   I. Title.
RM301.15.L48   1983   613.8'3   82–24951

ISBN: 0-07-037411-2
        0-07-037448-1 (PBK)

Book design by A. Christopher Simon

To my parents
DOROTHY AND MARVIN LEVY
whose nurturing and love
taught me the fundamentals
of life

To my loving wife JUDY
my daughter MERYL
and
my son DANNY
who are teaching the advanced
course

Contents

Introduction

Ours is a drug-taking society.

- 1½ billion prescriptions were sold in 1983 in American drugstores.
- Americans spend more than $1 billion per year on tranquilizers and another $1 billion on cold remedies.
- The pharmaceutical industry spends $1 billion a year on advertising (the liquor industry spends $100 million).
- $487 million from both public and private sources was spent for drug-abuse treatment nationwide in 1980 for some 260,000 drug-dependent people.
- Americans spend over $1 billion a year on over-the-counter (OTC) medications.
- The National Council on Alcoholism estimates that there are 15 million alcoholics and problem drinkers in America, with an annual cost to society in the neighborhood of $60 billion.
- Drunk drivers kill 25,000 men, women, children, and babies each year on American highways and injure 750,000 more.
- Over 20 million Americans have tried cocaine.

Americans do indeed have a love affair with chemicals.
In our attempts to understand this incredible phenomenon,

we have tried to define the problem in various ways. We speak of many dichotomies—licit versus illicit drugs, soft versus hard drugs, medicinal versus recreational drugs, mind versus body drugs, socially acceptable versus counterculture drugs—and invariably it all seems to fall into the ancient dichotomy "good versus bad." The use and abuse of all drugs is a very complicated affair with physical, mental, spiritual, economic, sociological, and anthropological elements. Polemics and rhetoric on all sides have only served to leave the lay public (and many professionals) in a state of confusion and what I call "rational paranoia" about most drug-related information. For example, concerning the great marijuana debate, Dr. Carlton Turner, President Reagan's White House Special Advisor on Drugs, graphically described this "opinion glut": "In six thousand papers I can support any conceivable idea you may come up with of what marijuana will do or what cannabinoids (61 of a total of roughly 360-odd chemicals in the plant) will do."

The sources of information, each one with its own set of biases, are often at odds with one another. Pressure is exerted on the individual by physicians, pharmacists, other health-care professionals, family members of all generations, friends and lovers (users and non-users), advertising campaigns by drug purveyors of every description, and the portrayal of drug use (with good and bad effects) in the entertainment industry. More and more people are being seduced by emotional appeals to join either the pro-use or the anti-use camp. Slogans range from "Better living through chemistry" to "Drugs are a cop-out." What is one to make of all these conflicting views? Jargonistic scientific reports, pseudoscientific claptrap, rigid and authoritarian pronouncements, all are presently competing not only for our hearts and minds, but for our pocketbooks as well!

This book is based on several premises which are designed to cut through the dense foliage of the drug jungle and clear a rational path to understanding:

1. Drugs have become an integral part of life in modern America.

2. Drugs are neither inherently good nor bad. All drugs have an abuse potential depending on who uses them and how.

3. We must assume full responsibility for what we put in our bodies, and conversely, we must not abdicate this responsibility to others.

4. A core of practical wisdom is already at hand to aid in making informed decisions about the drugs we use.

The main purpose of this book is to share with the reader some pragmatic concepts and caveats to guide you in taking on this personal decision-making process. Neither pro- nor anti-drugs, this book is *pro-health,* with a heavy emphasis on self-awareness, drug awareness, and self-control.

Health is defined here in a holistic context, that is, health as a positive state, not as the absence of illness. To the extent that drugs either enhance or diminish health, they deserve our serious and undivided attention. And in speaking about health, I place equal emphasis on physical, psychological, and spiritual components. Thus, the book is offered in the spirit of seizing control of our own lives and joining in a true partnership with professional experts and providers of health care. The late Dr. John Knowles, former director of Massachusetts General Hospital and Rockefeller University, in his thought-provoking volume *Doing Better and Feeling Worse—Health in the United States,* states:

> When all is said and done, let us not forget that he who hates sin, hates humanity. Life is meant to be enjoyed, and each one of us in the end is still able in our own country to steer his vessel to his own port

of desire. But the costs of individual irresponsibility in health have now become prohibitive. The choice is individual responsibility or social failure. Responsibility and duty must gain some degree of parity with right and freedom.[1]

This book is organized in terms of the various contexts and settings in which drugs of all kinds are used. The central theme, repeated in all chapters, is: *Drugs are not a drug issue—drugs are a people issue!* While specific information is supplied about a wide variety of prescription, OTC, pleasure, and other drugs (alcohol, nicotine, caffeine), the major emphasis is on the human context of drug taking. The book specifically avoids moralistic arguments, political rhetoric, and emotionalism. It is meant to be the eye of the hurricane. It will help you to understand how drugs are used and why; to test your own drug-taking behavior against some rational ideas concerning use and abuse; and will tell you how to handle difficulties without having to resort to outside help. It is not a book for addicts and alcoholics; many of those have already been written. It is a book for the lay person who is at neither extreme of either addiction or drug phobia. It is intended for the millions of Americans who every year cross back and forth over the shifting line between drug use and drug abuse and who need sound and reliable information to keep their lives in order. It is based on the principle that people are responsible for what they put into their bodies and that we are all in grave danger the moment we give up that responsibility.

Chapter 1 is about *drugs and the family* because this is where lifelong health attitudes and practices are first experienced. If parents wait for the fifth-grade science teacher to get to the drug curriculum it will be far too late. Families determine many patterns of behavior regarding drugs, and parents have the opportunity to teach moderation, to teach children how to deal with pleasure and pain, and to create a family setting in which free and open exchanges are possible. This chapter will help you and your children negotiate family rules about privacy, discuss drugs together, and set rational limits for drug-taking behavior. It will help you to define a drug problem, including alcoholism, and tells you how to help someone in your family who has such a problem. It discusses some common issues faced by families and suggests ways of dealing with them.

Chapter 2 deals with *drugs and school.* It will introduce you to the extent of student drug and alcohol use in America (it is quite high). The sometimes hazardous relationship between drugs and studying is examined, with suggestions for avoiding these hazards. It takes a close look at some tough issues like peer pressure, cliques, and popularity, and how drugs play a role in these matters. It contains a frank look at the risks involved in dealing drugs. It goes into some considerable detail about running a good school-based prevention program with suggestions for parental involvement as well as participation by students, teachers, and administrators. And it provides some direct guidelines for kids to help themselves and their friends who are having problems with drugs.

Chapter 3 is about *drugs and the workplace.* Drugs, including alcohol, are costing American business millions of dollars each year. In addition, we describe some of the less obvious but still dangerous kinds of drug use and abuse: nicotine, caffeine, smoking, and obesity. Many people fail to appreciate the profound impact these behaviors have on our health, our work mates, and our careers. Drugs and the world of sports is discussed. How companies can promote health in the workplace and the concept of employee assistance programs are described. You will be able to rate your own use of drugs and how they may be affecting you at work.

Chapter 4 deals with the subject of *drugs as medicine.* It helps you assess and appreciate your own role when it comes to dealing with the two people who should be your active partners, your doctor and your pharmacist. It contains specific advice about drug factors, patient factors, and physician factors—knowing what you are taking, why you are taking it, how to take it, dealing with side effects and adverse reactions, informing your doctor about all the drugs you are taking, drugs and pregnancy and breast feeding, storage and dating, contraindications, food and drink interactions with medications, limited activities, drug-to-drug interactions, stopping medications, drugs and your children, and drugs and older people. You will be warned about a phenomenon called the "dated" physician and shown why they are a problem for us all. There is a section entitled "Women Beware!" which speaks to sexism in drug-prescribing practices. The habit-forming nature of some medications is discussed, and alternatives to standard medical practices are suggested.

Chapter 5 is all about *getting high,* something that millions of Americans are doing every day. The high risks of adulterated and bogus drugs are described, and some advice is given on how to avoid these bummers. Cocaine is examined as the most seductive and expensive—in terms of dollars and risks—drug around. You will learn some of the serious cautions about methaqualone (ludes) and smoking and snorting heroin. Special emphasis is placed on the many hazards of various drug combinations, with particular attention to mixing drugs with alcohol. The seemingly mystical relationship between sex and drugs is examined and a list of drugs that enhance or diminish sexual functioning is included. Your awareness will be heightened regarding sane practices while partying with drugs so that you can have a good time without risking adverse reactions. You will be warned about the dangers of drinking, drugging, and driving, which can equal a prescription for death. And finally there is concrete advice about how to deal with adverse drug reactions when they do occur.

The appendices include an extensive table of commonly used drugs with their indications, contraindications, generic and brand names, street names, possible side effects and adverse reactions, psychological and physical dependence liability, and other information. There is a listing of sources of reliable drug information and literature, with information on finding treatment and self-help agencies across the country. There is also an annotated bibliography of supplemental readings. Lastly there is a listing of the marijuana laws for the fifty states.

By the time you finish this book you will be able to manage the drugs in your life. You will be able to more safely and intelligently integrate drugs into your personal health-care plan. You will develop a more mature and rewarding relationship with your doctor and pharmacist and a more assertive pro-health approach to pleasure drugs.

CHAPTER ONE

Drugs and the Family

The first three years of life form the foundation for all later development. Waiting until the fifth or sixth grade to educate children about the use and abuse of drugs can be disastrous. Parents must begin educating their children at the earliest possible moment.

Attention to the issue of youthful drug use has been overshadowed by a focus on peer-group pressure. Peer pressure *is* central to youthful experimentation with many things—sex, drugs, lawbreaking, outlandish dress styles—but we are neglecting, in a serious manner, attention to the earlier preteen years. Long before children feel the powerful influences of their friends, they are profoundly and indelibly affected by their immediate family. Young people enter their teens already influenced by parents, siblings, and other family members. It is difficult to bring about change later because patterns established in the earliest years of development persist throughout life and are resistant to change.

Family influences have been at work from birth, helping to shape and determine the young person's value orientations, knowledge and attitudes about drugs, feelings of self-worth, sense

1

of moderation, assertive behavior, ability to resist temptation, and body image. Parental emphasis on peer influence is often a cop-out and a smoke screen to hide our guilt and responsibility for our own drug-taking behaviors and the influence of these behaviors on our children.

Attitudes and beliefs about drugs start in the home, and they are effectively communicated to even the youngest member of the household. The family plays a vitally important role in early drug education, one which will help prevent or encourage problems with drugs later on in life.

EARLY EXPERIENCES WITH MODERATION

I took my family out to dinner at a local diner the other night. Seated two tables away from us was a family of four—all obese. My thirteen-year-old daughter was the first to notice them and pointed them out to the rest of us (my wife and ten-year-old son). I asked my kids what they thought of this sight, as the family proceeded to gorge on large desserts after an enormous spaghetti dinner. They were appalled by what they saw. My son said, "I'm glad you and Mom are normal and that we don't eat like that." I realized that by the example of our own physical appearance, the healthful manner in which my wife has fed our children since birth, and our own attitudes about overweight people, we had helped to teach our children about a very important concept—moderation. (Once in a while we will indulge in what the kids call "pigging out," but this is the exception.) As my wife and I discussed this incident in the diner we came to realize how, through a combination of "do as I do" and conscious attention to diet (and exercise), we had shaped our children's attitudes and behavior concerning moderation in food and drink.

The youngest children watch our behavior with fascination and bewilderment. They observe us at times when we are least aware of it. Like a child's version of *Candid Camera,* they will observe us as we grope around the kitchen until we have that first cup of coffee, they watch us light up a cigarette before we eat or brush our teeth, they see us pour a drink before dinner, they see Dad drinking beer in front of the TV set, they watch Mom and her friends sip cocktails at the luncheon, and they watch (depending upon parental guidance and censorship) an endless stream of drug-taking behaviors on television. They experience our lives in a very immediate way, and as they are already deeply emotionally involved with us (parents and siblings), our behavior registers in important ways. Young children learn, in part, by mimicking behavior. They love to imitate us. They put on our clothes, put Daddy's pipe in their mouth, play with an older sister's pompoms, and the like.

Families are powerful social systems where beliefs, opinions, ideals, and attitudes toward inner and outer reality are forged. Families generate their own "myths" much as in Greek or Roman mythology. These myths are a composite of all the belief systems created and reinforced by the family unit. By the time children interact with peers, the myths are firmly established and are accepted without question. Part of the family myth is that what one's own family does is "normal." What other families do that may differ is "deviant." As children interact more and more with the world outside the family, they test the power of the family myths. When their beliefs are challenged, these kids tend to dig in their heels and defend the family honor with a vengeance. But they remember what they have heard and seen and bring it home to us. In an attempt to sort out their own emerging personal sense of "normalcy" and "deviance" they ask us about our eating, drinking, smoking, and drugging behaviors. And this is where primary prevention starts. If we attempt to slough off these questions with vague or evasive answers, then it will be too late by the time the children reach the fifth-grade science teacher's unit on drug-abuse prevention. We as parents can effectively doom the curriculum years before it is taught in school. Kids are very sensitive to hypocrisy and lying in adults, especially their own parents.

Families can support and teach the important concept of moderation. Even in families where alcohol is regularly consumed, problems of abuse need not arise. There are entire cultures that have long histories of relatively safe drinking. They share certain drinking practices:[1]

- Children are exposed to alcohol early in life, within a strong family or religious group.
- Parents present a consistent example of moderate drinking.
- The beverage, normally wine or beer, is viewed mainly as an accompaniment to food.
- Drinking is considered neither a virtue nor a sin and is not viewed as proof of adulthood or virility.
- Abstinence is socially acceptable; excessive drinking or drunkenness is not.
- Alcohol use is not the prime focus of an activity.
- These "ground rules" of drinking are widely agreed upon by all members of the group.

The point is simple: if we model excessive behavior for our children, then we can not reasonably expect them to practice moderation.

Let's examine another area of human behavior where immoderation and compulsive consumption styles can lead to problems in youth and adulthood.

Barbara's Story

At age sixteen my son entered psychotherapy at my urging. He was forty pounds overweight and never participated in sports and had very little to do with girls. He was always eating. I thought it was because he had such a lousy self-image and was lonely. One day he informed me that his therapist wanted to see me. As a concerned mother I went to the session expecting to be asked purely psychological questions. Almost all of the therapist's questions had to do with my son's earliest eating behavior. I learned I had done it all wrong. He was my firstborn and I was never sure what he wanted when he cried. I always thought he was hungry when he cried, so I gave him a bottle which he gladly accepted and drank. I also found

4

out that I had started him on solid foods too early. The food made him thirsty, so then I would give him another bottle. I never dreamed that I was causing a problem which would emerge later on. Chubby babies are so cute. The therapist explained to me that what I had done was to help my son to learn that all or at least many of his discomforts could somehow be alleviated by eating. After all, I didn't just give him food and drink. I held him and kissed him and talked to him while I fed him. So food became associated with love and comfort and gratification. My son is now trying to sort out better ways to meet needs that food can't. I really thought I was doing the right thing at the time.

Barbara learned, in the course of her own psychotherapy, that she had confused her own needs for love and nurturing with eating and then transferred them to her son. This single case can help us to understand that eating behavior, in our society, involves a complex set of social and personal development circumstances. The expression "you are what you eat" tells only part of the story.

Body Weight Standards*[2]

The usual fat content of the body as a percentage of body weight is as follows:

American men	age 25: 14%
	age 55: 26%
American women	age 24: 25%
	age 56: 38%

Male trained endurance athletes usually have less than 12% fat. Female athletes have less than 18%.

Men are considered to be obese if they have more than 25% fat, and women if more than 30% fat.

* These are objective standards. Standing nude in front of your mirror may convince you that you are "fat." If you feel or look fat, then you are fat.

Fat children are likely to become fat adults. Both heredity and environment play a role. The "fat cell hypothesis" suggests that there are critical periods in early life when fat cells are formed. If excessive numbers are formed in response to overfeeding, the theory states, they become a lifelong problem. One study has shown that most severely obese people have too many fat cells, while more moderately obese people have too much fat in a relatively normal number of fat cells. Most experts support the theory to the extent that they strongly advise against excessive feeding during early life, particularly the first two years.

While we are not certain of the genetic linkage regarding heredity and obesity, we are aware of the statistical relationships. Dr. Jean Mayer[3] reported in his study in the Boston area that 7 percent of children of thin parents (or at least parents who were not overweight) were too heavy. If one parent was overweight, the proportion jumped to 40 percent. If both parents were overweight, the proportion reached 80 percent. Adopted children do not show this correlation. Overall, about one in eight schoolchildren in America are obese, and 58 percent of them will become obese adults.

Despite the compelling genetic evidence, the influence of the home environment is quite important too, and evidence is mounting which shows that adopted children mimic the behaviors of obese adoptive parents. The fact is that only about 1.6 percent of obese people are that way because of an underlying condition such as problems with metabolism or endocrine function. The rest have learned eating patterns that have led them into obesity.

Our earliest life experiences with eating have a profound effect on later behavior. At birth a baby lives and loves with its mouth. The sucking response in infants is necessary to life (whether the mother employs breast or bottle feeding). How the mother and the father hold the baby during feeding is important. Both parent and baby must be relaxed for feeding to be a pleasurable experience. During the act of feeding a complex series of behaviors occur from which parent and child clearly derive benefits other than the simple transfer of nutrients. Tender words, warm physical contact, a reassuring presence; all of these contribute to emotional well-being and the experiencing of eating as enjoyable. According to Erik Erikson: "The oral stages, then, form in the infant the springs of the basic sense of trust and the basic sense of mistrust which remain the autogenic source of both primal hope and of doom throughout life."[4]

Listed below are some hints for getting your children to eat in a healthful manner.

- Set an example. Eat nutritious foods, avoid junk food, and eat reasonable amounts. Eat with your kids, especially breakfast.
- Know what your kids are eating both in the home and outside and how much they are consuming.
- Avoid sugar-laden products in the home. Check labels of cans and boxes. You'll be surprised how many food-stuffs have added sugar. You can't blame kids for eating such foods if you buy them.
- Substitute healthy snacks. Experiment with different items until you find the ones that your kids like and will eat.
- Educate your kids. Take them with you to the supermarket and let them experience comparison shopping both for pricing and nutrition content.
- Help your kids to acquire good eating health habits. Most food preferences are acquired. My kids didn't even know about sugar in cereals, added or processed, until they were much older. By then they had already developed a taste for unsweetened grain products. The same applies to salt (again read labels and model the appropriate behavior).
- Water, fruit juices and milk are good for you at any age. Soda is not something that is part of a nutritious diet. Especially if you want to avoid sugar and caffeine. Explain the importance of vitamins and minerals.
- Don't be afraid to set up rules and guidelines for family eating behavior. However, avoid rigidity because it invites cheating. You may even want to allow periodic "pig-outs" where everyone "cheats" within reasonable limits.

Compulsive immoderate eating has many parallels with compulsive immoderate use of drugs and directly threatens individual and family health.

DEALING WITH PAIN

Life is filled with pain, both physical and psychological, in so many forms: physical illness, mental illness, loss, separation, rejection, criticism, accidents, poverty, racism, sexism. The list is endless. Some pain is acute, that is, sudden and short-lived; some pain is chronic in nature, tending to persist over long periods of time. How we deal with pain is a central issue, as pain, like stress, is unavoidable. Our children look to us to shelter them from pain and to reduce or eliminate it when it occurs. One of the surest ways that life engenders both humility and frustration is in forcing us to realize that we can not ultimately protect our loved ones from pain. A whole new science of pain management is presently being developed, which includes such things as biofeedback, electrical and chemical brain stimulation, autogenic and relaxation training, and meditation. Freud was right in his notion that we are guided by a pleasure principle and seek to avoid pain.

One of the ways that people have sought to pursue pleasure and avoid pain is through the use of drugs, including prescription, over-the-counter (OTC), and so-called illicit or street drugs. A patient of mine who underwent radiation therapy for a cancerous condition described his experience:

> After each treatment I was subject to severe nausea and vomiting. It was so awful. I would vomit until my stomach was empty and then go into dry heaving. My psychologist suggested the use of THC [tetrahydrocannabinol] as an anti-nausea drug. In my case, the THC really helped reduce the nausea and vomiting. The THC had only one side effect—I got stoned!

The radiation treatment was necessary to prevent cancerous tissue growth. The THC (one of the active chemicals found in the marijuana plant and extracted in the laboratory) reduced the side effects associated with the treatments and induced a pleasurable altered state of consciousness. (There are still many states where THC can't be legally prescribed for this purpose. Patients are advised to discuss this treatment with their doctors, as THC doesn't appear to work in all cases.)

Here is another example of drug use to avoid pain:

> My life is one hassle after another. Constant demands from my job. More demands from my kids when I get home. Make dinner, supervise homework, mediate fights. And then my husband wants me to be loving and alluring after the kids go to bed. Thank goodness for my Valium. I don't know how I would get through the day without it.

This woman was suffering from the "superwoman" syndrome and was trying to be all things to all people. Rather than face the basic issues, she retreated into the daily use of a tranquilizer meant for episodes of acute anxiety and stress. While Valium was never intended to be a "maintenance" drug (taken daily), this woman was experiencing pain on a daily basis in the form of anxiety and tension. Therapy consisted of facing the superwoman trip and renegotiating family roles with her husband and kids. Goodbye Valium, hello family support!

And a final example from a very unhappy patient:

> DR. L.: How long have you been experiencing the mood swings you just described?
>
> PATIENT: All through my adolescence and most of my adult life. I'm now thirty-seven.
>
> DR. L.: What kind of treatment have you received before coming to me?
>
> PATIENT: Ten years of group and individual psychotherapy! All to no avail!
>
> DR. L.: How has it been since you started taking lithium [carbonate] prescribed by Dr. Z. [a psychiatrist]?
>
> PATIENT: Well, once you and Dr. Z. helped me to see that I was suffering from manic-depression, I have been

taking my lithium faithfully for three months. I can't tell you how much better I feel. The mood swings are less volatile and my life at home is much happier.

This patient, suffering from a major psychological disorder, manic-depression (or bipolar illness), experienced no relief from his psychic pain by means of talk therapy alone. Without the lithium therapy he was doomed to suffer from an illness which is not under conscious control.

Pain is a symptom which alerts us to the fact that something is not right with ourselves or our world or both. Sometimes the source of the pain is internal and sometimes it is brought about by an external agent. When we take drugs to alleviate pain we often create a psychic state which further prevents us from taking our own inventory to determine the source of the pain. Not knowing or otherwise avoiding the source, the best one can hope for is symptomatic relief—and this can be achieved only by repeating the use of the drug. People facing interpersonal difficulties are the best example of this vicious cycle. Failure to identify and cope with the source of our difficulties can lead to a dilemma: an unresolved problem *and* a drug problem. For example, while many people enjoy using drugs and alcohol for recreational purposes, there are those folks who can't function around other people *without* drugs. The issue is not the drugs so much as the inability to socialize. Here are some "trigger" questions to help you determine how you deal with pain:

- When I hurt, do I feel that I have to tough it out (machismo or machisma) and suffer in silence?
- When I hurt, do I live with the fear of what might be causing the pain or do I check it out with others (family, friends, professionals)?
- Do I consider it unmanly or unwomanly to cry?
- Do I worry about my image and pretend all is well?
- When I hurt, do I bottle it up until I feel like exploding (or actually explode)?

- Do I tend to minimize my pain? maximize (exaggerate) it?
- Do I run to the medicine cabinet?
- Do I use alcohol to alleviate my pain?
- Do I believe that drugs are magic and will make everything okay?
- Do I make an honest appraisal of my situation and try to figure out what is causing my pain?
- Do I believe that I deserve my pain?
- When I know the source of my pain, do I deal with it directly?
- Do I accept pain as a part of life?

One of those aspects of personality which is central to an understanding of how we deal with physical or psychic pain is the disparity between our true self and our image. We all develop an "image" which we use in a conscious manner to impress other people. In our more honest private thoughts we sense a truer self, free of the constraints of our image, a sort of personal bottom line. This is our irreducible essential self. The fears, ambitions, jealousies, strengths, and weaknesses reside here. Sometimes the distinctions between the image and the true self become blurred. The greater the disparity between the true self and the image, the less likely we are to handle pain well and to turn to "artificial" means such as drugs to cope with pain.

Here is a simple exercise you can do to see how aware you are of these distinctions. Take a sheet of paper and draw a line down the middle. Label the left-hand side "my image" and the right-hand side "my true self." Several categories are suggested in the example. These headings are neither good nor bad, just different. List all the traits, attributes, or behaviors that rightfully belong in each column.

Once you have completed the list, you can decide what value to place on the two listings. People who use a lot of drugs have a tendency to live in the world of images more than in the world

Category	My Image	My True Self
friends	I am close to people.	I have trouble trusting.
	I enjoy people.	I'm basically a loner.
sex	I can take it or leave it.	I enjoy sex a lot.
	I'm a real lover.	Women (men) scare me.
feelings	Nothing bothers me.	I'm easily hurt.
	I'm very sensitive.	I use tears to manipulate people.
money	I'm doing real well.	I'm insecure about money.
	Money is unimportant.	Money matters a lot.
power	I'm in charge around here.	Who's really running things?
	I'm not afraid of anyone!	Pushy people scare me.

of the true self. Most relationships are image-to-image. Real friendship and love relationships bring us more into a "core-to-core" orientation. One of the reasons you use drugs may be either a sense of discomfort with your true self or too many image-to-image relationships, which leave one feeling empty. Only you can know for sure. The more you live within your image and the more discrepant the image from the true self, then the more you will fail to handle pain in satisfying ways. Self-honesty is the best route to dealing with pain and discomfort. You are freer to be honest with others when you can break through your image. Sharing pain is one of the best ways to break through.

Within the family context we adults model ways of dealing with pain for our children. If they see us seeking chemical short-cuts instead of squarely facing issues and going through the difficult task of resolving them we have given them a poor example of facing up to reality. From a holistic point of view, when a family member is in pain (of any origin), he or she is suffering on a physical, emotional, and spiritual plane. These planes of experience cannot be separated. There is an emotional component to all physical illness, and physical upsets affect us emotionally. The spiritual area may involve a sense of God or an existential reality or simply our own sense of mortality. We are rapidly learning how loneliness, for example, contributes to the aging process. When you are in pain you need to be healed. Families that can share pain, share feelings, and reach out to their members can heal pain. Families that alter painful reality with drugs alone end up with a dual problem—the original problem plus a drug problem. After a while the two become indistinguishable and pain becomes chronic. Chronic pain requires chronic drug usage! If, as parents, you model the "macho" approach, then don't be surprised when your kids don't share their pain and troubles with you. They are simply feeding back your own behavior. If you pop pills or booze to deal with your problems, don't be surprised when your kids mimic this. You have taught them that this is how your family deals with pain. And when taking prescribed medications to alleviate pain and suffering, take them as prescribed, don't change doses on your own, report side effects to your doctor, and be alert to the effects of combining several drugs. For more on this issue, turn to Chapter 4.

DEALING WITH PLEASURE

We may put the question whether a main purpose is discernible in the operation of the mental apparatus; and our first approach to an answer is that this purpose is directed to the attainment of pleasure. It seems that our entire psychical activity is bent upon procuring pleasure and avoiding pain, that it is automatically regulated by the pleasure principle.[5]

Very few people would disagree with Sigmund Freud's notion that we seek to avoid pain, but how to pursue pleasure has always been the source of bitter debate. From the hashish-smoking Sufis of ancient Arabia to the pot-smoking hippies of the 1960s; from the drunken revelries of Roman bacchanals to the fraternity and sorority beer blasts of modern times, people have sought out pleasure in the form of drugs of every conceivable description. It is true that there are societies in which certain chemical pleasures are forbidden: alcohol to the Muslims and Mormons, grass and cocaine to the devotees of the "moral majority." How your family defines pleasure and permits or forbids its pursuit will have a profound impact on family attitudes and behaviors regarding drugs. If you were to ask each member of your family to make a list of positive and negative human emotions, you would quickly discover that the negative list is almost twice as long as the positive list. Life is filled with enough pain for us to have developed a vocabulary that reflects this aspect of what we commonly call reality. The pleasure principle is counterbalanced by what Freud called the reality principle. The reality principle also seeks pleasure—but it is a delayed and diminished pleasure, tempered by the harsh facts of life. Chemicals allow us break through delay and pain and can take us to the heights of pleasure, ecstasy, and corporal delights. Disputes about pursuing pleasure via drugs cut deeply into personal belief systems, and often battle lines are drawn along generational lines. Listen to one family attempting a discussion in this volatile area.

> SON (AGE 17): When I get high [on grass] I explore parts of my mind and soul that I can't reach any other way. It's like I go more deeply into myself and find both joyous and frightening things. I love being touched when I'm high, and conversations with other people become easy.
>
> FATHER: Someone your age has no business using drugs. When I was your age I was already out working. There was no time for such foolishness. You had better explore your mind by concentrating on serious matters like school.
>
> MOTHER: You should be able to enjoy life without drugs. You don't see me using drugs or alcohol to have a good time. You're just looking for kicks. All you kids today have it too easy.
>
> SON: You don't understand! I take care of my schoolwork and my part-time job. I'm looking to go beyond these simple facts of my daily existence. I'm searching for a higher consciousness—something greater than myself.
>
> MOTHER: You can find that in church!

SON: God is within me as well as without. There are many ways to seek Him and grass does that for me.

FATHER: You spend too damn much time trying to feel good. Who said that life is full of good times? You will have to work hard just like my father and I.

Embedded in this conversation are some bedrock beliefs held by the parents which mitigate against their own pleasure seeking and are projected onto their son. Their statements are heavily value-laden and reflect a rigidity that prevents them from hearing their son. Perhaps the son will have it easier than the parents, working less and playing more. His parents seem threatened by this and, worse, seem embittered in a way that closes off understanding and communication.

Part of the problem is simply that what pleases one person is not necessarily pleasurable to another. One person's pleasure may be another person's idea of pain. But the fact remains that drugs make people feel good or at least ease the way to good feelings. As adults we may seek to deny our children access to certain physical and psychic pleasures, but we can be sure that their friends will tell them about it. Kids are into pleasure and have not yet made bargains with life which call for delay of gratification.

Church and state have sought to govern and regulate the pursuit of pleasure throughout recorded history. Lay and religious laws and precepts have been laid down to control and suppress certain forms of pleasure, most notably alcohol and drugs. In many instances puritanical beliefs have allowed laws to be passed that defy reason and scientific credibility. Harry Anslinger waged a one-man antimarijuana campaign that led to the creation of such laughable products as the film *Reefer Madness,* which depicts the "killer weed" as the source of unbridled sex and violence. No one doubted his sincerity, but his exploitation of the issue may have contributed to pot smoking more than it diminished it.

Among their recommendations, the editors of *Consumer Reports* in their book *Licit and Illicit Drugs* list the cessation of scare tactics and the proper classifying of drugs; moderating two counterproductive aspects of Harry Anslinger's approach. Marijuana to this day is listed by the federal government in the same category (called Schedule I) as heroin and morphine (both narcotics).

In 1970 key federal legislation, Public Law 91–513, the Comprehensive Drug Abuse Prevention and Control Act, was enacted into law. The first major change in the federal law since the Harrison Narcotic Act of 1914, it is more commonly referred to as the Controlled Substances Act of 1970. Various drugs are listed in five categories, called schedules, primarily according to medical usage and abuse potential; the most dangerous in Schedule I, the least in Schedule V.[6]

Schedule I

A. The drug or other substance has a high potential for abuse.

B. The drug or other substance has no currently accepted medical use in treatment in the United States.

C. There is a lack of accepted safety for use of the drug or other substance under medical supervision.

Includes heroin, hallucinogens such as mescaline, LSD, psilocybin, and marijuana. Use is forbidden except for highly restricted research purposes.

Schedule II

A. The drug or other substance has a high potential for abuse.

B. The drug or other substance has a currently accepted medical use in treatment in the United States or a currently accepted medical use with severe restrictions.

C. Abuse of the drug or other substance may lead to severe psychological or physical dependence.

16

Includes opiates and synthetic opiates such as morphine, metha-done, and Demerol, certain barbiturates of the short-acting type, methaqualone, cocaine, and amphetamines. In this schedule, pro-duction quotas may be set, import-export quotas are imposed, and telephone and refillable prescriptions are prohibited.

Schedule III

A. The drug or other substance has a potential for abuse less than the drugs or other substances in Schedules I and II.

B. The drug or other substance has a currently accepted medical use in treatment in the United States.

C. Abuse of the drug or other substance may lead to moderate or low physical dependence or high psychological dependence.

Includes Doriden and Noludar 300, barbiturates, and paregoric. No production quotas, looser regulations, and no prescription re-strictions except prohibition of refills after six months.

Schedule IV

A. The drug or other substance has a low potential for abuse relative to the drugs or other substances in Schedule III.

B. The drug or other substance has a currently accepted medical use in treatment in the United States.

C. Abuse of the drug or other substance may lead to limited physical dependence or psychological dependence relative to the drugs or other substances in Schedule III.

Schedule V

A. The drug or other substance has a low potential for abuse relative to the drugs or other substances in Schedule IV.

B. The drug or other substance has a currently accepted medical use in treatment in the United States.

17

C. Abuse of the drug or other substance may lead to limited physical dependence or psychological dependence relative to the drugs or other substances listed in Schedule IV.

Schedules IV and V differ little from Schedule III and from each other. Schedule IV includes long-acting barbiturates such as phenobarbital, Placidyl, and chloral hydrate, and minor tranquilizers meprobamate, Librium, and Valium (manufacturers contested the inclusion of the latter two). Schedule V includes cough medicines with codeine with certain age restrictions.

There are many controversies surrounding what schedule a particular drug or class of drugs is included in. For example, some of the tranquilizers included in Schedule IV have shown themselves far more dangerous in terms of addiction and withdrawal than marijuana, which is listed in Schedule I and has no known physical addiction or established withdrawal syndrome.

While you may agree that laws are needed to control dangerous substances and their distribution, we should all understand that what really is at stake is the legislation of morality. All drug laws exist because powerful members of our society have been able to influence the legislative process to enable government to regulate the pursuit of pleasure. Judging from the fate of Prohibition and the extent of the drug traffic in America today, we are not doing too well in this area. This has prompted some to call for dispensing with all laws prohibiting drug use. The National Organization for the Reform of Marijuana Laws (NORML) is working toward the removal of prohibitions against marijuana. (For a listing of existing marijuana laws on a state-by-state basis, see Appendix D.) The editors of *Consumer Reports* and the former Drug Abuse Council (sponsored by the Ford Foundation) have been among those groups calling for a more rational re-examination of drug laws. At the other end of the spectrum are groups like the Texans War on Drugs, the American Council on Marijuana, and the National Federation of Parents for Drug-Free Youth. These groups seek harsher drug penalities, the establishment of antiparaphernalia laws, and ultimately the cessation of all illicit drug use. Antiparaphernalia laws are probably sitting on constitutional quicksand, because their definitions of drug-using materials tend to be vague. No matter what side you take in these issues, you can be sure that the law of supply and demand will overshadow all else. Ancient and modern history has shown repeatedly that when people want drugs they find ways to get them, and the supply may ebb and flow but it never stops. We have yet to articulate a rational national policy on drugs. The legal one—alcohol—is the leading drug of abuse, even though regulated by the government. The illegal ones are controlled by organized crime. Why we sanction some intoxicants and not others does not seem to be founded on scientific facts. Rather it is the issue of legislating pleasure that is at the heart of this whole controversy. Alcohol influences consciousness as surely as marijuana and cocaine do, and yet we do not think of alcohol as a drug. We have a long way to go in sorting out these issues.

In the meantime, here are some "trigger" questions to help you and your family determine how you conceive of and deal with pleasure.

- Do I consider the pursuit of altered states of consciousness a legitimate pastime in seeking pleasure?
- Do I consider it okay to pursue these altered states with drugs?
- Do I use chemicals to make me feel good? Can I do this without guilt feelings?
- Are words like ecstasy, delight, sweetness, orgasmic, and pleasure-seeking part of my personal vocabulary?
- Is the pursuit of pleasure for its own sake okay with me?
- Am I open to exploring new means of seeking pleasure?
- Do I explore new horizons of pleasure in areas like sex?
- Do I look down on people who seek pleasure in ways that differ from my own?

- Do shame and guilt prevent me from enjoying my life? In what areas?
- Do I have good reasons for allowing or disallowing the people I love to experience pleasure?
- Do I allow myself to feel good?
- Do I feel I always have to be "in control"?
- Do I believe that I deserve to feel pleasure?
- Do I have good reasons for delaying gratification?
- Do I project my own values onto other people, or am I open to what they say and do?

Once you have taken a hard look at how you handle both pain and pleasure, you will be ready to consider other areas such as privacy and limit-setting with less of a risk of hypocrisy or confusion.

PRIVACY

Privacy is one of those terms that everyone thinks they understand until someone's privacy is invaded. Then, in that moment of heat and anger, the parties realize that they may have very different conceptions of just what privacy really is. If you think that all members of your family share a clear agreement about issues of privacy, try this simple test. Tonight, around the dinner table, ask each person to define the term. You go last. Have someone act as recording secretary and write down everyone's definitions and notions. Don't be shocked if there is some real divergence of opinion. By raising the question, you have set the stage for one of the most important issues your family may ever have to face. How does this relate to drug usage? Consider the following aspects of privacy in situations involving drugs.

Controlling access to spaces: "John and I were smoking a joint in my room. My father came in without knocking. I caught hell for smoking dope, but I was furious because he doesn't even respect me enough to knock. I have no rights in my own room."

Controlling access to information: "At dinner last night my parents grilled me for a half-hour about who among my friends is drinking and using drugs. What a drag. I know they are concerned about me, but what my friends do is none of their business."

Being alone: "My wife went off to her usual card party on Thursday night. I finally had a chance to try that piece of hashish that Terry gave me. Well, about three hits into a great head my wife came home early. She did not feel well. She doesn't dig drugs. There went a great high."

Personal property: "I believe that my room and the stuff in it is my personal property and that I have a right to my privacy. Whether it's ludes or condoms, I don't want my mother going through my things. I don't want to have to be paranoid in my own space."

The message about drugs and privacy is that all four of these dimensions have one important and powerful element in common: social control. Whoever controls these various aspects of privacy controls the family unit and its goings and comings. All parents attempt to control their children, and as the children get older, they in turn try to exercise some control over their own lives and the lives of the adults around them. With older children, this attempt to control has a double edge. The parents call the shots; they set down the rules and set limits for the children. The children, on the other hand, can either comply or circumvent the rules.

Privacy can be found in all cultures and societies. There is even major evidence of "privacy" behavior among many species of animals. The need to exercise the freedom of privacy is vitally important to all Americans. As a society we have many concerns about the invasion of privacy by, among other people or groups, the press, the government (federal, state, local), the school system, computers, the clergy, law-enforcement agents, the banks, the credit card companies, and the Internal Revenue Service. We jealously guard our privacy but we rarely define it, negotiate it, and discuss it within the family unit. It usually comes down from parents by direct or indirect fiat. There is one phrase that children abhor hearing their parents speak: "Who ever told you that you could ———!" If you often find yourself saying that, on any variety of topic, it is a strong clue that limits have not been clearly established.

There are parents who, in the name of love and concern, come down very hard on the issue of privacy. They honestly believe that by exercising tight control they can prevent their children from getting into "trouble." Here trouble is defined as doing anything the parents don't like. This works up to a point. If the kids find you inflexible and rigid, they will scheme to get around you. The more you attempt to deny them their privacy, the more their behavior will become secretive; they will "go underground," drugs in tow. The trouble with denying people privacy is that they can turn around and do the very same thing to you. How? you might ask. Let's say you control space and information. You can't keep your kids under constant surveillance no matter how much you "bother them." They can cut off much of their communication to you. Then everyone begins living in separate and narrow corridors within your home. But there are some things you can do, together with all members of your family, to work out this very sensitive issue.

How to Set a Framework for Privacy Within the Family

- Let everyone know that this important topic is going to be discussed. Get a consensus for a time and place free of intrusions. Be prepared to spend more than one session at it before everything is worked out.
- Everyone is going to enter into the discussion with preconceived notions. The first ground rule is that nothing will be decided until everyone has had a chance to be heard and some discussion has taken place.
- A good starting point is to have everyone define "privacy." The next step can be to have each person state his or

her concerns about the presence or absence of privacy for them in the household.
- Be sure to cover all four primary areas in the discussion:
  1. controlling access to space
  2. controlling access to information
  3. being alone
  4. personal property
- Once you reach the point where decisions are being made and rules established, write them down, reproduce them, and distribute them to all members. This "contract" on privacy is open to amendments and changes. However, another meeting should be convened before the rules are changed.
- Everyone should be prepared to state his or her rationale for suggested rules. Statements like "because I say so" don't help anyone. Yes, parents may have the ultimate say, but it should not be for arbitrary and capricious reasons.
- While it is not necessary to spell out what will happen each and every time the privacy contract is violated, there should be some notion about redress of grievances. This might start with another family conference. Remember, one member's behavior can have an impact on all other members.

The secret to having this work out well is the willingness of the adults to really involve the kids. Then it's up to everyone to deal with the issue in good faith. No magic here, just something that seems to have disappeared in many families: mutual communication and respect.

TALKING ABOUT DRUGS

In some ways this whole drug thing is like the weather. Everybody talks about it but no one can do anything about it. That's because most of us get lost in sociological generalities, have strong

23

emotional biases, and don't bother to check out the facts. We feel compelled to come down strongly on one side of the issue or the other and to join a camp that has already articulated its position: *Drugs Are a Cop-Out! Better Living Through Chemistry! If You Need a Drink to Be Social, That's Not Social Drinking! Turn On, Tune In, Drop Out! Why Do You Think They Call It Dope? Feed Your Head! Take It Easy! Reefer Madness!* Generalizations and oversimplifications. The whole issue of drug use is complicated and multifaceted, yet users and nonusers alike feel compelled to make extreme statements. People write off each other's views for reasons like "you can't trust anyone over 30," "they don't get high," "he works for a drug treatment program," "he's a cop," and so on. Amidst all the rhetoric and emotionalism, when the National Institute on Drug Abuse announced a few years ago that the U.S. government was cooperating with the Mexican government in spraying Mexican marijuana fields with a deadly herbicide called paraquat, pot smokers began checking their ounces for black burn holes (caused by the paraquat). And with good reason, because paraquat-adulterated marijuana can cause serious pulmonary problems. Between the government's high visibility, public-relations–minded attempts at modifying consumption, and unscrupulous dealers selling the poisoned grass, the consumer is caught.

The most important thing about education (in public schools, private schools, churches and synagogues, camp, the home) is the development of a "learning attitude," an attitude of openness to new information from all sources, a willingness to hear what others are saying, the courage to examine unpopular views, to look at the minority view, and to make up your own mind.

Hints for Parents on Talking About Drugs With Your Children

1. You don't need to be a drug expert to hold a discussion with your kids, only a concerned parent. However, it is a good idea for you to get your drug facts straight (check out resources at the back of the book). Your kids may be able to share informational resources as well.

2. Be honest about your own drug use. Remember, caffeine, nicotine, and alcohol are all powerful drugs. This is an area where many families get into deep trouble. Kids are very sensitive to hypocrisy.

3. All drug experiences teach us something about ourselves. Listen to your kids before reacting.

4. When laying down rules of expected behavior (i.e., no "hard" drug use—no pills, no opiates, no speed), be clear and up front. Don't be wishy-washy and don't make threats you are not prepared to follow through on.

5. Know before you get into this discussion just how much of your own private life you wish to reveal.

6. If you don't want your kids to use certain drugs until they reach a particular age due to differences in physical and emotional maturity, state your case.

7. Don't grill your kids about their friends. You should ask what the local youth drug scene is like, but don't play grand inquisitor when it comes to your children's friends. They will tell you what they think it is important for you to know (usually what they are anxious about).

8. Don't fall into the trap of thinking that all is well if your kids are just drinking. Alcohol in its many forms is just as dangerous as any other drug. Drinking doesn't mean they are not using drugs. Lots of kids do both (so do adults).

9. Try to avoid stereotypes. For example, by conservative estimate, two-thirds of the high-school class of 1981 had tried at least one illicit drug in the year—but that doesn't mean *your* kid did.

10. Recognize that part of being young and growing up is being curious about many things including drugs, pleasure seeking, establishing an identity, copying other kids, rebellion against authority, and the like.

11. The fact is that all you can really do is share your feelings and concerns, state some ground rules and sanc-

tions, and then stand back. You can guide, but you can't really control.

12. Let your kids know that if they have a problem with drugs, any problem, you want them to come to you for help.

13. Remember that drugs are used in a context, and the context can be as important as the drugs themselves.

Since two-way communication is the goal, here are some traps to avoid.

Don't:

    lecture and preach
    forget to listen
    interrupt a lot
    be condescending
    be arbitrary and capricious
    mistake passion for reason
    yell a lot
    exaggerate or lie
    be hypocritical
    insult their intelligence
    refuse to have future discussions on the subject

Good luck!

SETTING LIMITS

Life is full of "shoulds," "oughts," and "have-tos." Children learn them from parents, siblings, friends, teachers, religious leaders, and other authority figures. It starts out with "Thou shalt not" and often ends up with "You'll do it if you know what's good for you!" But here in the United States we value and cherish individual freedom of choice. True, there are some groups, religious fundamentalists foremost among them, who would restrict

26

these freedoms and have us all live our lives according to their narrow interpretation of "right living." The vast majority of Americans, however, will defend to the death their right to individual freedom. Parents reserve the right to raise their children as they see fit, and as long as they don't violate the law, they can exercise this right to govern the lives of their offspring.

Juxtaposed to this parental guidance is a necessary and important fact of life: the only love relationship that must, by definition, lead to separation is the love between parent and child. All other love relationships bring people closer together. Your children, in order to grow into their own maturity, must begin moving further and further away from your parental supervision and influence, until one day they make the physical break with home. We accept this as the natural order of things.

But somehow when it comes to the subject of drug use, our love and concern become tinged with fear and ignorance. We imagine the worst, seeing pushers lurking in schoolyards ready to force drugs upon our children. (The fact is that most kids get their drugs from their friends.) We try to protect our kids by any means possible. We lecture, threaten, cajole, promise, beg, plead, intimidate, and all manner of authoritarian hell tends to break loose. Just about all kids (starting in fifth or sixth grade) will be exposed to the youth drug culture, and most will sample the wares at least once. If primary prevention means never trying a drug, then we as a nation have failed miserably in this regard. I think we must place our emphasis on secondary prevention. That is, accepting that most kids will try drugs, we must help them to not risk toxic or lethal drug effects. This process starts with an honest appraisal of the whole issue of setting limits. Let us begin by stating a maxim: *Parental authority is never absolute!*

You may choose to go to the ends of the earth to see that your children obey you, but when it comes to the assertion of their emerging individuality, "never say never." They will find ways to evade you. Any kid can beat any parent at this game! The harsher and more persistent your exercise of authority, the cleverer and more devious their efforts to thwart you. Once it gets this far, both parent and child are in a lot of trouble anyway. One of my adolescent patients says:

> My parents are very strict. They really laid down the law about drugs, sex, friends, you name it. I am afraid of them. Every time I tried to talk to them about how hard it is being different from my friends, they would rant and rave and threaten me. I started keeping vodka in one of the beakers in my chemistry set in my room. Vodka has no real odor and I figured the best place to hide it was in plain sight. They never caught on. I felt bad about sneaking, but it serves them right for never listening or trying to understand.

It may not be terribly clear to many kids and even to some parents why any limits concerning drugs are necessary. Explore how each member of your family feels about the reasons listed below and you will get a better sense of what the limits need to be in your family.

Why Kids Need Limits Around Drug Use

1. Many drugs are illegal, and so is underage drinking. Getting arrested and/or having parents called down to the station house is a real bummer for everyone concerned. No one needs an arrest record following him or her throughout life.

2. Peer pressure is very hard to resist. By laying down limits you help your kids to stay "in bounds." When friends pressure them to drink or drug, they can say things like "If my parents see me with red eyes [or funny-smelling breath, or slurred speech], I am going to be grounded." They may still have to deal with being called "chicken," but no real friend would lay that trip on them.

3. The use of drugs is fraught with danger, and I don't mean just addiction. Lots of adults and kids get into

28

trouble (bad trips, drunkenness, fights, accidents, etc.) in a single episode of intoxification. Limits help reduce the dangers.

4. Drinking, drugging, and driving don't mix, and parents are wise to be most assertive on this issue.

5. Limit setting is part of loving when you are a parent. No limits is as bad as too many limits.

6. Many drugs are adulterated or misrepresented (ersatz speed that is really caffeine, ludes that are really Valium, grass laced with PCP or paraquat), and even your best friend can't tell you if he or she doesn't know about it.

7. Parental limits will help your kids to develop internalized limits (which may be exactly the same or may differ). They need a starting point, which is your job as a parent. Their developing experience and maturity will take over from there.

A Rational Guide to Limit
Setting Between Parents and Children

Do:	**Don't:**
Set a time and place for what will probably be a lengthy discussion.	Treat this issue lightly.
State the limits clearly and in objective terms.	Be vague.
Make sure the kids are direct parties to the setting of these limits. Put some faith in them.	Forget that kids resent arbitrary authority and will cooperate more readily if they "own" part of the process.
Give yourself and your kids a sense of trust in their ability to deal with these issues.	Predict doom or expect perfect compliance all of the time.

Do:	Don't:
Realize that the purpose of limits is to guide, not to control.	Think your authority is absolute. You won't be there when they try drugs.
State your fears and concerns as parents and take a position on the issues.	Fail to set some limits. Kids need them, and none is as bad as too many.
Try to get a sense of how kids and parents in your community are dealing with the drug issue.	Worry about keeping up with the Joneses. Set limits that meet your family's needs.
Make any sanction clear.	Say one thing and do another.
Be prepared to change the limits based on actual performance; be flexible.	Set them down in concrete.
Realize that if your kids are in trouble, they need your help.	Give up your authority to any outside agency (police, other parents, etc.).
Advise your kids to say nothing without advice of counsel if they are arrested.	Seek to punish before you know the facts. Believe your kids.
Set reasonable limits based on drug facts.	Lump all drugs together (and remember that alcohol is a drug).

There are kids in some families who will violate limits continuously and otherwise fail to respond to parental authority or standards of reasonable behavior. It is important for all children to learn that their behavior has consequences. When kids rebel and repeated efforts, including professional intervention, prove fruitless, then a more radical approach may be called for. One method for dealing with these most difficult situations is a program called Toughlove. Developed by David and Phyllis York, Toughlove's logo is a heart with a clenched fist, and the program draws a tough line indeed. Problem teens are told to "shape up or ship out," meaning to conform to acceptable standards or literally leave home. That is the tough part about Toughlove: a parent must be prepared to say to the youngster, "You have to choose between living in our family as a decent human being or leaving." Kids are not thrown out on the street; they are given the option of staying with friends, relatives, or other Toughlove parents. An important part of the program is the support given to parents by other parents in the Toughlove network. Before presenting your child with this hard decision, make sure you have tried all other avenues and sought professional counseling and advice. For information on Toughlove, see Appendix C.

ABOUT ALCOHOL

I can't tell you how many times over the years I have heard parents say "Thank God my kid only drinks and doesn't do drugs." *Alcohol is a drug!* It is the most popular social drug in America and it is also the most abused (the National Council on Alcoholism estimates that there are 10–13 million adult alcoholics and problem drinkers in the United States). Alcohol is a sedative, or depressant, drug with many properties and actions similar to the barbiturates (which are also sedatives). One of the worst addictions is a combination of pills and booze since the effects are superadditive. One study showed that, used with alcohol, a nearly 50 percent lower dose of barbiturates was lethal than when the drug was used alone. Alcohol has no nutritional value but loads of "empty" calories.

In case you still don't want to think of alcohol as a drug, let me make a comparison between alcohol (Ethanol or ethyl alcohol) and a substance everyone agrees is a drug—heroin. There is no evidence of any long-term damage to the human body from years and years of heroin use. Oh, of course, you can get hepatitis from dirty needles, die from an overdose of the drug, or get shot trying to steal a television set (heroin addiction is a nasty lifestyle). But the heroin itself does not hurt the body. It is metabolized and completely broken down. Now, what happens when you drink a fair amount of booze (comparable to a daily heroin habit) on a regular basis? Well, you see, ethanol can invade any cell in the human body and cause short- and long-term damage to any organ system. You can go from a fatty liver to alcoholic hepatitis to cirrhosis (where liver cells atrophy and die), or you can go from short-term memory loss (blackouts) all the way to Korsakoff's disease (alcohol amnestic disorder). And that's just the medical side. The psychological and emotional problems associated with alcoholism and alcohol abuse are equally awesome.

People develop a tolerance for alcohol. Scientifically, this occurs because of the brain's adaptation to increasing levels of alcohol. Behaviorally, what it means is that over time it takes more of the drug to get the original effect. People who become physiologically addicted to alcohol experience withdrawal when their supply is suddenly cut off or drastically reduced (the same is true for heroin). This withdrawal reaction is typified by elevated temperature, pulse, and heart rate, plus sweating, nausea, disorientation, and fear. The "d.t.'s"—delirium tremens—are the same as withdrawal, only much more exaggerated. Both conditions need to be treated in a hospital setting. *Alcohol is a drug—a powerful sedative drug which must be treated with respect!*

Here is one sad story that makes the point very clearly:

> We enjoyed an open and honest relationship with our son Michael. He came to us when he was seventeen and said that a lot of the kids were getting into drugs and that he was frightened by this. We suggested that perhaps if he were to limit his own behavior to just alcohol he could deal with the peer pressure. Michael thought this was a good idea and even told us that it worked quite well. He just told his friends he preferred to drink while they smoked marijuana or took other drugs. Around graduation time the kids were partying a lot. Michael asked if he could use the family car to take his date and several other kids to the prom. We happily said yes. After all, he had shown

us that he was a sensible and trustworthy person. The night of the prom, at around two A.M., we received a call from the police. Michael and the other kids were involved in a car accident. One child was dead and the others injured seriously. Miraculously Michael received only minor injuries. When we arrived at the emergency room the police informed us that Michael was being arrested for drunk driving. He had drunk the equivalent of a pint of vodka and a half a bottle of champagne. Celebration turned into tragedy. Six years later he still wakes up screaming in the middle of the night and blames himself for what happened. And we thought we had given him some good advice when we said it was okay to drink. How could we have been so blind? Alcohol is just as dangerous as any other drug!

Here are answers to some frequently asked questions about alcohol that may aid you in discussing this subject within your family.

Q: Alcoholics are those bums on skid row. Why should my family worry about it?

A: Only about 5 percent of the estimated 10–13 million alcoholics and problem drinkers in America can be found on skid row. The rest are people just like you and me.

Q: I heard there are no Jewish alcoholics.

A: This is an excellent example of a powerful but false stereotype. The recent work by the Task Force on Alcoholism and Drug Abuse in the Jewish Community of the Commission on Synagogue Relations of the Federation of Jewish Philanthropies of New York has shown this to be untrue. When Drs. Sheila Blume and Dee Dropkin conducted their study of one hundred Jewish alcoholics, they found one A.A. group in New York City that had forty Jewish members. And that was just 1 out of 1300 meetings held in the greater metropolitan area each week. No one is sure about the actual numbers, but alcoholism occurs among Jews, and the time for denial is over. There are many Jewish people in Pills Anonymous (P.A.) as well.

Q: I heard that alcoholism runs in families. Is that true?

A: Many professionals believe that what we call alcoholism is a disease for which there is no known cause or cure. There is some interesting and compelling evidence that leads us to believe that there may be a genetic component, but there is no real definitive proof. Statistically, we know that if one parent is alcoholic, the offspring have a one-in-four chance of developing alcoholism. If both parents are alcoholic, the odds increase to one chance in two. However, there are alcoholics with no family history of the disease.

Q: What happens if you give some coffee to someone who has had too much to drink at a party?

A: The best you can hope for is a wide-awake drunk! It takes the body 1 to 1½ hours to metabolize one drink (12 ounces of beer, 5 ounces of wine, 1½ ounces of whiskey, one highball or cocktail) to the point where there is no accumulation of alcohol in the blood. The caffeine in the coffee will act as a stimulant but cannot counteract the depressant aspects of the alcohol. Cold showers and walks in the night air don't help either. Only the passage of time—as I said, about 1 to 1½ hours *per drink*—can do the trick.

Q: How much alcohol is too much?

A: An alcoholic is someone whose drinking causes a continuing problem in any department of his or her life. For the chronic disease, the key word in the definition is "continuing." For any single episode of drinking, a person is in trouble when his behavior causes a problem for himself or the people around him. This definition doesn't get hung up with how much, how often, or what form the alcohol comes in. All that matters is that when you drink things go wrong. The most important question you can ask someone for whom you have a concern is, "Has anyone ever spoken to you about your drinking?" A positive answer may indicate a drinking problem, and the matter should be pursued further.

Q: Is it true that it's okay for kids to drink beer or wine? Isn't it the hard stuff that causes problems?

A: Alcohol is alcohol, no matter what form it comes in. Beverages differ in their alcohol content: beer and ale contain 3 to 6 percent, wine contains 12 to 14 percent, and hard liquor contains 40 to 50 percent (80 to 100 proof). Problems are caused by drinking too much alcohol no matter how it is packaged. There are alcoholic beverage products that are marketed to look like anything but alcohol (usually containing a lot of sugar). This is an attempt to capture the youth market. All states have laws that prohibit the sale of any alcoholic beverage to those under a certain age. These laws exist because the use of a powerful drug like alcohol needs to be controlled. The official judgment is that kids under the legal age are not mature enough to handle it.

Q: How does someone know when there is a real problem with alcohol in their life?

A: Here are some questions that can help in making a self-assessment (you can substitute the term "drug" for "drink" to test yourself regarding other drugs):

1. Do you usually drink heavily after a disappointment, a quarrel, or when the boss gives you a hard time?
2. When you have trouble or feel under pressure, do you always drink more heavily than usual?
3. Has a family member or close friend ever talked to you about your drinking behavior?
4. Have you noticed that you are able to handle more liquor than you did when you were first drinking?
5. When drinking with other people, do you try to have a few extra drinks when others will not know it?
6. Are there certain occasions when you feel uncomfortable if alcohol is not available?
7. Have you recently noticed that when you begin drinking you are in more of a hurry to get the first drink than you used to be?
8. Do you sometimes feel a little (or very) guilty about your drinking?
9. Did you ever wake up on the "morning after" and dis-

cover that you could not remember part of the evening before, even though your friends tell you that you did not "pass out"?

10. When you are sober do you often regret things you have done or said while drinking?

11. Are you secretly irritated when your family or friends discuss your drinking?

12. Have you tried switching brands or following different plans for controlling your drinking?

13. Do you often find that you wish to continue drinking after your friends say they have had enough?

14. Have you often failed to keep the promises you have made to yourself about controlling or cutting down on your drinking?

15. Do you lose time from work due to drinking?

16. Do you often have trouble performing sexually after drinking?

17. Have you ever tried to control your drinking by making a change in jobs or moving to a new location?

18. Do you try to avoid family or close friends when you are drinking?

19. Do you eat very little or irregularly when you are drinking?

20. Do you sometimes have "the shakes" in the morning and find it helps to have a little drink?

21. Do you get terribly frightened after you have been drinking heavily?

22. Have you recently noticed that you cannot drink as much as you used to?

23. Do you sometimes stay drunk for several days at a time?

24. Sometimes after periods of drinking, do you see or hear things that aren't there?

25. Have you ever been in a hospital or institution because of drinking?

If you answered "yes" to between one and three of these questions, you should carefully consider whether or not you have a drinking problem. If there were four to seven "yes" answers, you should consult an alcoholism expert and discuss the negative role alcohol is playing in your life and what to do about it. Eight or more "yes" answers indicate that you are in serious trouble and should seek treatment services immediately.

DEFINING A DRUG PROBLEM

One of the difficulties in defining a "drug problem" is that it depends on who's doing the defining. Perceptions differ radically within the same family unit, in much the same way as in the tale of the four blind men examining an elephant—each one declares the part he touches to be the definitive beast. Here are some terms defining levels of drug involvement to help us get started.

Experimentation: The first experience or two with a given drug.

Drug use: Periodic or regular use of a drug. No ill effects to self or loved ones.

Drug abuse: Any frequency of usage which leads to ill effects to self or loved ones.

Drug addiction: Compulsion, negative life consequences, and loss of control define addictive process. Physical and psychological dependence are consequences of chronic drug usage. Physical addiction component defined by establishment of tolerance and appearance of withdrawal symptoms upon cutback or stopping. Preoccupation with drugs as a way of life.

The difficulty arises out of one's effort to further define "ill effect." We tend to be very egocentric about these matters. For example, the answer to "How do you know when you're doing too much drugs or alcohol?" is often "When you're doing more

37

than I do!" "Which drugs tend to cause problems?" "The ones I don't use!" One person's "problem" or "ill effect" is not readily agreed upon by others. I believe that the core of this issue is the denial and other ego defenses that people use to twist and distort what is going on. Here are some examples of how these defenses work:

Denial: "I do not have a drug problem." (But others think you do.)

Rationalization: "Everyone else is doing it. Why shouldn't I?" (Because you can't handle it.)

Compartmentalization: "I know I have blackouts, but I can handle my booze." (Person denies connection between events.)

Projection: "I don't need to use drugs all the time. You do." (Person attributes unacceptable behavior in him- or herself to others.)

Displacement: "It's okay for my husband to smoke pot, but I'll kill my kids if they do it." (Fear of husband causes target to be shifted.)

Sublimation: "Who needs those girls anyway? I'd rather go drinking with my friends." (Sexual motive is denied and replaced by socially acceptable alternative behavior.)

Intellectualization: "I only smoke filtered cigarettes, Mother, so there's nothing to worry about." (Denies feelings in oneself and others, very similar to rationalization.)

Since many of these defenses involve unconscious motives and feelings, do not expect people to see the light just because you bring it to their attention. Remember, they are defenses against disturbing information or insights.

Another important aspect of defining a drug problem is to realize that some problems are acute, that is, have a rapid onset and short duration; while others are chronic, usually building up over time and then persisting over time. Both can be either mild or severe. A person who has been through a "bad trip" on a hallucinogenic drug like marijuana or LSD can tell us a lot about the horrors of an acute drug reaction. A child who suffers from the lifelong effects (chronic) of brain damage caused by sniffing airplane glue has a problem of a very different kind. Some negative effects wear off as soon as the drug is completely metabolized (broken down chemically by the body), while others persist because of the damage done while we were using the drug. A person with a hangover pays some dues for the previous night's drinking, but a man who loses his arm in an industrial accident because his judgment was impaired by alcohol pays dues the rest of his life. Some drugs persist in the body for several days, like the THC in marijuana, while others are more short-lived, like alcohol. (By the way, although the THC remains in the body, the "high" lasts only a few hours at best.) What's interesting about drug storage in the body is the effect it may have when you use the same drug again. Science has a lot more to learn about this aspect of drug use.

Another important distinction must be made between a problem or problems preceding the use of drugs and those caused by the use of drugs. While it is certainly true that most people who use drugs do so to party, there are those who use them for other reasons. (Here I am not referring to the proper medical use of drugs.) Many different drugs have the ability to take us away from ourselves and our physical and emotional upheavals. They transport us, temporarily, to less painful states. The business executive hooked on Valium, the teenage pothead, the hidden-alcoholic housewife, the street junkie, the luded-out party freaks are all trying to flee problems in their lives through the use of drugs. In these cases there are pre-existing problems of loneliness, impotence, damaged egos, rejected loves, poor body image, family upheavals, anxiety, depression, and so on. They all have something else in common: using drugs is not the answer to these problems.

The two human conditions most frequently encountered in drug-abusing and addicted populations are depression and anxiety. For these people, drugs provide a stopgap. At best it is only a temporary haven, for when the drugs wear off, the problems are still there. For many, they now have two problems—the original one and the added drug problem. Drugs are only vehicles or means for traveling. They are not an end in themselves.

Parents often ask me to list for them those special things to look for so they will know when their kids are using drugs. I always give two responses to these inquiries: (1) ask the kids directly, and (2) almost all the symptoms that drugs can cause can be brought about by other situations and events. For example, some people tell parents to look for sudden changes in the kid's behavior, such as the quiet kid who becomes outgoing or the outgoing kid who suddenly becomes withdrawn. Drug use? It could just as easily be a hundred other things besides drugs (mood swings are common in adolescence). Another example: the kid starts spending more time in his or her room. Drug use? Try privacy, homework, phone calls to friends. If your child smells like a six-pack, staggers, has blazing red eyes or slurred speech— these are more likely to be signs of actual drug use. I've heard people say that you should look for needle marks. Well, if things have gone that far then you have been missing a hell of a lot about your kid besides drug use. Do you think that anyone knows your child and his or her behavior patterns better than you? Of course not! Don't look to the "experts" to do your job for you. Talk to your kids; ask them; tell them of your concerns for them. You should have been doing this all along. And not just when you think they are playing around with drugs. You should query your kids about anything in their behavior that confuses or upsets you. Drug problems are *people problems* and should be dealt with as such. Only people can fill that void— not drugs.

A person with a drug problem is someone whose use of drugs (including alcohol) causes either an acute or a chronic difficulty for himself or for the people who care about him. Determining that a problem exists is just the beginning. You may still have a problem in dealing with the defensive posture of the drug user. The main point here is that you should be prepared to confront the person directly and honestly with an account of how their drug-taking behavior is affecting you. Also be prepared to state your concerns about what drugs may be doing to them. Stay open to the possibility that the "problem" may be yours and that the two of you may never really agree about the fine distinctions between drug "use" and drug "abuse."

If you want to know how drugs figure in your own life, stop taking them for some significant period of time, like a month or two. (Do *not* stop taking prescription medications without the advice of your physician.) If you are concerned about the effects of stopping nonprescription drugs, check with a knowledgeable professional. See how you do without the drug during this drug holiday. Here are some things to look for:

- Do you miss the drug?
- Are you experiencing any withdrawal effects? (If they get heavy, check with your doctor.)
- Does life seem less full without the drug?
- Are you suddenly aware of problem areas in your life that you had been ignoring?
- Are you having less fun without the drug (in bed, at parties, etc.)?
- Are you feeling tense or anxious?
- Are you feeling depressed?
- Do you feel better without the drug?
- Do you have problems concentrating or meeting goals and deadlines?
- Do you find that you spend a lot of time thinking about the drug?
- Did you put aside a stash just in case you missed it too much?

If your responses to these questions during your drug holiday have caused you some concern, then you should turn back to the section on alcohol and answer the twenty-five questions listed there. Getting more nervous about the drugs in your life? Perhaps the time has come to ask whether you can deal with this issue on your own. If you can't return to the drug with a clear conscience regarding your own health and well-being, then you may have a drug problem. If the conflict is so great that you find the decision weighing heavily in your life, something may be out of balance. Drugs can be used in many ways. Once they become the centerpiece of your existence, there is no doubt that something more vital may be missing from your life. Friends, a good self-image, a decent job—something is missing. You can throw all the drugs you want into that void—it will never be filled. You are probably looking for the right thing (love, respect, belonging, success) but in the wrong place.

HOW TO HELP SOMEONE IN YOUR FAMILY WHO HAS A DRUG PROBLEM

Rule #1: Don't deny the problem. You are in a unique and intimate position to see what is going on with your family member. Avoiding the issue is the worst thing you can do. Very often you can see clearly what the drinking or drugging is doing to the other person, but can you see what it is doing to you? The longer you join in the denial, the worse the problem can become. You are not responsible for the other person's drug use, nor are you responsible for their abstinence. You *are* responsible for your own feelings and reactions. Responsibility can be defined literally as the "ability to respond." Let yourself and the drugging person know that you are affected by their behavior.

Rule #2: Check out how this drug problem is affecting the entire family. Here is a story that makes the point: I once had a staff member who at the age of eleven was sitting on the front stoop of her house with four of her friends on a snowy November day. In the distance the girls could see a man staggering down the street and occasionally falling into the snowbanks. They all found this to be an amusing sight. When the man got closer to where they were sitting, the girls recognized him as the father of my staff member. They picked him up and helped him into the house. He reeked of alcohol. This was the last time she ever had her friends over to her home. The stigma of an alcoholic father led her into isolation and made the family home a taboo place to bring friends. *Everyone* in the family is involved to a greater or lesser extent when someone has a drug problem. The problem is felt in such ways as use of time, space, money, role distribution, arguments, attempts to protect younger members of the family, privacy, power, allocation of family resources and the like. Not sure how the problem is affecting you? Attend a meeting of a self-help group like Alanon or Alateen or Pillanon to hear how people just like yourself have been and are being affected by a drug abuser in the family. It will be an eye-opening experience.

Rule #3: Helping the family to cope is as important as helping the person with the drug problem. I have seen entire families destroyed by one member's serious drug problem. This does not have to be the case. You should hold a family conference without the drug abuser present. Let everyone acknowledge, each in their own way, how the problem is affecting them and how they feel about it. After the initial shock and denial, it is common for feelings of anger and resentment to come to the surface. You will all need each other, and children, including young children, should not be left out. There is more at stake than whether or not the abuser will be able to recover. Younger members of the family will be watching, for example, to see how the parents cope and how they respond to their needs. You must not neglect the rest of the family by pouring all of the family's resources into the abuser.

Rule #4: Realize that feelings are running high and try to come up with a rational plan of action. One approach to the issue which has been helpful in dealing with denial is the process of objective confrontation. At the family conference mentioned above, you can plan to confront the abuser. The rules are: (1) stay calm—emotional exchanges only lead to more defensiveness;

(2) present objective evidence of the abusive behavior (episodes of intoxification, failure to carry out roles, evidence of accidents, broken promises, etc.); (3) ask the abuser to listen patiently and not to defend his or her actions at this time; (4) state how this problem is affecting each of you as a family member; (5) state your willingness to support the abuser; (6) state the limits of this support; and (7) be prepared to offer resources. If you find that this kind of forum cannot be accomplished in your own home, then you can seek the help of an outside professional to guide your family through this process.

Rule #5: Labeling doesn't help. You want the abuser to get to an expert who can help him or her figure out what the problem is. Since denial and the other ego defense mechanisms mentioned earlier are so powerful, you cannot reasonably expect the abuser to buy what you are saying just because you say it (or even present objective evidence). You don't have to label the abuser an alcoholic or an addict (or a head, or a junkie). But you should state your concern and strongly suggest that the individual seek professional advice to sort out the nature of their actual problem. If they refuse, then you have some additional presumptive evidence for the extent of the problem.

Rule #6: Spell out the limits of how far the family is willing to go in supporting the abuser. Make sure the sanctions are clear. I refer you back to the section on limit setting. If the suggestions made there do not work out, then you need to seek outside help to accomplish this. There are growing numbers of family support groups that you can turn to (Alanon, Alateen, Pillanon, Toughlove, to mention a few). Check with local government or private programs to secure referrals of this type. A family has a right not to permit the behavior of one individual to ruin the quality of life for all its members. It really helps to get the support of your own peers to accomplish this difficult task.

Rule #7: You should carefully consider who the actual patient is. It may be the drug abuser or it may be the entire family. One member's drug abuse may be symptomatic of underlying problems within the family as a whole. On the other hand, the abusive behavior may be independent (in the main) of the family dynamics. The best way to tell is to seek out the services of a mental-health professional (psychologist, psychiatrist, clinical social worker) whom you know to be well versed in the area of families and substance abuse. Let this person aid you in forming a plan of action that takes three things into consideration: (1) the needs of the abuser, (2) the needs of the family, and (3) the possibility that the abuser is unwilling to seek treatment. Remember, people use drugs for a reason, and sometimes the reasons reside within the family structure. Whether this is the case or not, the abuser will need family support in his or her recovery, and the family must decide how they wish to accomplish this. Sometimes, in their need to punish the abuser, family members, parents in particular, refuse to consider family-oriented treatment. This is a shame because it means the prognosis will be poor, particularly for young people who must remain at home until they are old enough to leave.

Rule #8: People with drug problems have broken lots of promises. The best way to help is to deal with actual behavior. Action does speak louder than words. Whatever approach is chosen, the acid test (no pun intended) is how everyone actually lives up to their end of the bargain. Progress should be determined by objective criteria (homework done, treatment sessions attended, abstinence accomplished, curfews kept). Other family members will tend to distrust the abuser. The best way to overcome this is for the abuser to win back their trust through realizable goals and actions.

Rule #9: Don't get hung up with your family's image. Helping the abuser and your family are far more important than any stigma and embarrassment you may feel. Once you realize you have a drug problem in the family, you must understand that what is happening to your family is not unique. This problem is occurring all over America. It happens in the best of families and in the worst of families. It is happening to all kinds of folks in a very democratic fashion. Anyone is eligible—the rich and the poor; blacks, whites, Hispanics, Native Americans; educated and uneducated; men and women (boys and girls); families with histories of drug problems and families where there has never been a problem. Use your energies for resolving the problem at hand, not worrying about what your neighbors think. Everyone gossips anyway, so why worry? Your priority is your family. If the stigma is really getting to you, seek out people with similar problems (through self-help groups and drug treatment programs). You will be amazed how many "peers" you have. You need to know you are not alone. And you need to know that these things do happen to "people like us." The harder a family tries to cover up a drug problem, the more exposed they become anyway. Your family, friends, and neighbors are getting hipper all the time. So don't waste valuable energy and time trying to look good by denying the situation. Look good by having the courage to face the problem squarely.

Rule #10: Nothing can be accomplished if the abuser continues to abuse drugs. Drug counseling is the first order of business. When a patient comes to see me (youth or adult) with a drug problem, I consider it my responsibility to marshal resources to help this person stop abusing drugs. Drug abusers do not have the luxury of waiting for the doctor to figure out the answers to the "why?" questions. They could end up dead while the therapist tries to sort out their id, ego, and superego problems. Simply stated, the first order of business is to stop or reduce the drug taking. After this is accomplished, then more insight-oriented types of therapy can be brought to bear. Choose a therapist who has experience with your family member's type of drug problem. Ask lots of questions—it's a right, not a privilege. You don't need arrogant doctors during a drug crisis. Most people can stop abusing drugs without understanding all the reasons why they began or continued to use them. But the treatment must be geared toward this approach. If the prospective therapist or agency thinks months of therapy are needed to understand and deal with the drug problem before drug taking stops, go to another agency or practitioner. The folks in Alcoholics Anonymous (A.A.) have said it best: "First Things First."

SOME COMMON PROBLEMS FACED BY FAMILIES AND HOW TO DEAL WITH THEM

The Great Marijuana Debate

This issue tends to be very divisive. Within families it usually breaks down along generational lines. A lot of things have been attributed to marijuana that scientific research doesn't support. The most objective statement that can be made is that marijuana is not an innocuous drug. Most people use it without ill effect. A few people have a severe negative reaction called a marijuana psychosis, which is a toxic reaction similar to an allergy. Certainly for this minority the drug is anything but innocuous. There are studies that show damage to fertilized mice ova, changes in the brain cells of rhesus monkeys, and a number of similar reactions in a variety of animals. The fact is that no one yet knows the long-term effects of occasional and heavy marijuana use in humans. There is some evidence that there are even more carcinogens (cancer-causing agents) in marijuana smoke than in that of conventional cigarettes.

The definite answers are not yet in, and pro- and antimarijuana forces quote those studies which best support their bias. A 1982 report on marijuana and health released by the National Academy of Sciences states:

> Our major conclusion is that what little we know for certain about the effects of marijuana on human health—and all that we have reason to suspect—justifies serious national attention.

In 1982 the American Medical Association and the U.S. Surgeon General warned users of grass that it is not a harmless diversion free of harmful effects. Basing its position on twenty years of

47

published scientific research, the Public Health Service has concluded that marijuana has "a broad range of psychological and biological effects, many of which are dangerous and harmful to health." The harmful effects or suspected effects include:

- Impaired short-term memory and slow learning
- Impaired lung function similar to that found in cigarette smokers
- Decreased sperm count and sperm motility
- Interference with ovulation and prenatal development
- Impaired immune response
- Possible effects on heart function
- By-products of marijuana remaining in the body for several weeks with unknown consequences. The storage of these by-products increases the possibilities for chronic effects as well as residual effects on performance even after the drug has worn off.

It is best to keep in mind that, as I've emphasized before, all drugs have an abuse potential and if mismanaged can cause ill effects. While some drugs carry an outright danger in any amount of use, others may require repeated use before harmful effects are noted. For example, you are far more likely to get sick to your stomach from your first snort of heroin than to experience any ill effects from your first joint of marijuana.

So you see the scientists can't give us definitive enough evidence about grass to tilt the scales in either direction. That means we have to look at it from other perspectives. One of the ills reported to be associated with marijuana use in the young is something psychiatrists have named the "amotivational syndrome." According to this theory, marijuana use causes lethargy and listlessness— the young people neglect their studies, withdraw socially, and lose all ambition. Antimarijuana groups are fond of quoting this one. However, it must be remembered that adolescent drug abuse is a complicated and multidimensional problem. For every kid who may show the signs of this so-called syndrome, there are many thousands who give no evidence of it whatsoever. A teen-

48

ager who loses all ambition and ceases his studies is indeed going through some kind of crisis. However, rather than the crisis being caused by smoking grass, it is far more likely that it is causing the drug use and the kid is "self-medicating" with grass, which can act as a mild antidepressant. He is using this otherwise recreational drug the same way a psychiatrist would prescribe some antidepressive medication: to counteract feelings of sadness or loss. Again, the problem is not the grass he smokes as much as the situation, internally and externally, that has led him to seek this chemical release. Most kids I've worked with or treated who use grass this way have other nonchemical pressures weighing heavily upon their lives. Once I have helped them to clearly identify the root problems and to face them, the drug abuse diminishes and the school performance (or other educational or vocational choice) improves. The social withdrawal always stems from poor self-image and some actual social rejection. It isn't easy for many of the young to break into the tight cliques that form during the middle and high-school years.

I was on a panel recently where the usual assortment of liberal and conservative viewpoints were being expressed by my co-panelists. When a kid in the audience asked about the apparent hypocrisy surrounding adult use of alcohol versus teenage use of marijuana, one of the speakers said, "Every time you light up a joint the purpose is to get high, while an adult taking a drink has no intention of getting high." He fell right into the trap that the questioner had laid for him. Both marijuana and alcohol are mood-changing drugs. How high you get does depend, in part, on how much of the drug you consume. But it's hypocritical to state that one is taken to alter one's mood while the other is not. Caffeine and nicotine cause changes in mood as well. Ever run out of cigarettes or coffee? So let's at least be honest about the comparisons we make.

The bottom line on the issue of marijuana, as it is for many other drugs, is the effect the drug has on your life and functioning when you take it. Simply taking a toke on a joint is not evidence of drug abuse. Suffering ill effects and wishing to repeat the behavior is drug abuse. Persistence of drug use in the face of serious disruption of functioning is psychological addiction. This can happen with marijuana, but it is still the exception, not the rule. What is the effect of marijuana (and its chemical sisters—hashish, hash oil, THC extract) on growing minds and bodies? No one is sure. Can marijuana affect unborn fetuses? Again, no one is sure, but it's wise not to smoke *anything* when you are pregnant. We once did not think alcohol could be harmful to unborn children, but we now have clinical evidence of fetal alcohol syndrome (FAS) which shows that drinking during pregnancy can lead to serious problems for the child. Chemicals of all kinds seem to be able to cross the placental barrier. The taking of all drugs carries a calculated risk. In the absence of clear and definitive scientific pronouncements about marijuana, you are well advised to exercise caution and moderation. Millions of people will have no one to blame but themselves if grass turns out to have some as yet unknown negative surprises. There is no intended scare tactic in these statements—just an emphasis on the judicious exercise of common sense and the acceptance of personal responsibility for your own health and the health of your loved ones.

What if It's the Parents Who Are Abusing Drugs?

As adults we usually emphasize the perils of adolescent drug abuse. Here the shoe is on the other foot. For example, there are 13 million adult alcoholics and problem drinkers in America. Many of them have children. In New York it is estimated that 9.4 percent of the state's children have an alcoholic in the family. We do not make nearly enough of an effort in supporting and guiding these children. Here are some ways in which these children are affected and actions they may need to take when their parents are involved in serious drug abuse.

It is not their fault. Kids have a way, when their parents are in trouble, of thinking that somehow they are the cause of the problem. This can occur with marital discord and breakup, child abuse and neglect, and drug abuse. The kid thinks, "If only I had been a better son [or daughter], if only I had behaved better [or done my homework on time, or gotten better grades], or . . ." Kids are not responsible for their parents' drinking and drugging. And they are certainly not responsible for their sobriety. These are choices that adults make for themselves. Kids have to learn to detach themselves from these unfounded guilt feelings and focus on managing their own lives.

Kids must not deny the impact of parental drug abuse. The parents' behavior is probably making them feel scared, helpless, and angry. The parents have probably become unpredictable, making and breaking promises, spending less time with them than before, ranging in their moods from loving attention to callous disregard. There may even be improper sexual attention or advances from parent to child. There may be unexplained beatings or punishment. The kids go through terrible conflicts about their own vacillating feelings of love and hate toward a parent. They begin losing respect for the parent; this is confusing and frightening. These kids need to be brutally honest with themselves about their own feelings, however conflicting or negative they may be. Repressing these natural reactions will only cause more damage. These youngsters are forced to grow up too fast as they ride the emotional roller coaster created by parental drug abuse.

The children need to talk to their parents. One of the reasons that some adults persist in their chemical abuse is that they can fool themselves into believing that they are not harming their families. The children must let the parents know how their behavior is affecting them and how they feel about it. The parents need to know that their children are worried about them. If only one parent is abusing drugs, then the children should speak to the other parent. Kids need to know that you share their perception of what is happening to your partner. They need to understand what is happening to the family. They must not be shut out—drug abuse is a family problem.

Kids must learn not to try to run their parents' lives. It is quite common when one or both parents are in trouble with drugs for the children to seek out a form of role reversal in which they try to care for the hurting adult(s). They begin assuming more responsible roles within the family, plugging gaps and trying to maintain a semblance of normalcy. This tends to bring childhood to a screeching halt and forces kids to grow up too fast. In an effort to hold things together, they may turn into superachievers in school and at home. What the kids really need to do is to lead a parallel existence, in which they take care of their own responsibilities and are not dragged down by the parental behavior. If things get too crazy at home, they need to spend time in the school library or at a friend's house. Seeking out self-help groups like Alateen can be very helpful and supportive in the kids' efforts to keep their own lives together even as their parents may be going to hell in a bottle (or syringe or whatever).

There is a real danger that children may begin using drugs themselves in an effort to punish their parents. The parents have already set an example of "better living through chemistry" and the kids follow in kind. I have worked with families where there has been drug abuse in three generations—children, parents, and grandparents. The real danger is that the kids may find temporary relief from their own bad feelings by using drugs. If this happens they will begin seeking that relief on a regular basis. The fact that the parents may do it with booze while the kids are doing it with other drugs is of no consequence. Getting high is getting high, regardless of what drug is taken.

Kids become isolated and feel terribly embarrassed by their parents. Remember the story of my staff member who, once it became known that her father was an alcoholic, never again invited her friends to her home (she was only eleven years old at the time). Children of drug abusers feel a powerful stigma and are subject to profound feelings of embarrassment. Their own homes become off-limits because they never know when their own parent(s) might do something to cause them to feel ashamed. Even worse, they may stop feeling worthy of their friends and retreat into a lonely world where their only friends exist in their fantasies. These kids are desperately in need of a real friend—

someone they can talk to, dump their feelings of fright, anger, and confusion on, and get emotional support from. It is embarrassing to admit that a parent is in trouble with drugs, but it's even harder to go it alone. These kids don't need their friends to have answers, just for them to be there for them when they are hurting.

Even after the kids have done everything in their own power to cope with a bad situation, they may find that they need professional help. It isn't easy to "keep on keeping on" when you are alone and confused. Younger children may approach a favorite teacher or guidance counselor. Older ones may seek out a psychologist, social worker, or psychiatrist. It's a great relief to these kids when they find a confidant who can guide them. They need to know that theirs is not the only family facing this problem. The professional should guide them toward new peers such as those in groups like Alateen or Alanon. The worst thing is for the kids to feel compelled to go it alone and be crushed by the overwhelming pressures of a family in serious trouble.

According to Sharon Wegscheider, who works with the families of alcoholics, the children learn to adopt what are described as "survivor roles." Four of these are described below:

- The family hero. Often the oldest child, he or she works extremely hard at gaining family approval. Usually an overachiever who wants to please, he or she becomes the family's representative to the outside world.
- The scapegoat. Feeling emotionally rejected, this child uses defiance to strike back at the family. A lot of negative energy is focused by the family on this antagonistic child who provides a focus that keeps attention from the drinking parent.
- The lost child. The lost child learns to avoid close relations within the family, spending a lot of time alone or quietly busy. He or she suffers from intense psychological pain and loneliness. The pain is often masked by the apparent self-sufficiency and independence.

- The family mascot. Often the youngest child in the family, he or she is not taken very seriously, mostly due to age. Often hyperactive and may use humor or obnoxious behavior as a means of getting attention.

The Clean Air Act: Smoking at Home

There is growing evidence that exposure to smoke from another person's cigarette may be harmful to the health of nonsmokers (the same holds true for pipe and cigar smoke). There are two kinds of smoke emitted from a burning cigarette. Mainstream smoke is that portion of the smoke drawn directly from the mouthpiece of a tobacco product (pipe stem, cigarette tip with or without a filter, end of a cigar) during active puffing. Sidestream smoke emits from the smoldering tobacco in a steady stream. Smoke particles and various smoke ingredients are found in sidestream smoke in even higher concentrations than in mainstream smoke. Passive inhalation is the involuntary taking in of this sidestream smoke (together with exhaled smoke) by a nonsmoker. People with allergies (including asthma) are more sensitive to this smoke than others. We can't yet definitively state that passive inhalation causes cancer, but future epidemiological studies may prove this to be the case. Here are some nonmedical reactions to parental smoking from a group of fifth-graders I spoke with:

I don't kiss my father anymore. I can't stand his breath!

My mother's hair and clothes smell like an ashtray full of dead butts.

We stay far away from the family room on football-game days. The smoke makes my eyes water and makes me choke.

It makes me angry that both my parents can smoke in any room in the house. The whole house stinks from cigarettes. Don't I have a right to some clean air?

Last weekend I threw my mother's cigarettes in the garbage. She just went out and bought some more. My father told her that she is addicted and she threw an ashtray at him.

I told my mother and father that they are not allowed to smoke in my room anymore.

If you believe that you are actively promoting good health in your home, you had better consider this issue if anyone in your family smokes any tobacco product. At the very least you are polluting the air. At the very worst you may be actively endangering the health of your loved ones.

The Clean Air Manifesto

1. Stop smoking. If you can't, reduce your tobacco intake at home.
2. Keep your smoking limited to as few rooms in the house or apartment as possible.
3. Try to keep your smoking to an absolute minimum when other people are around.
4. Keep the windows open.
5. Make a conscious effort to keep more square footage between yourself and other people (not too effective without proper ventilation).
6. Respect the rights of nonsmokers of all ages.
7. Ask your guests to keep their smoking to a minimum (or if you have stopped, ask them not to smoke at all in your home).
8. Do not smoke at all around infants and toddlers.
9. Do not smoke in your children's rooms.
10. Consider giving it up again. It's for your own health as well as your family's.

By the way, smoking in your car, because it's a smaller space, is even worse. The smell of smoke lingers in a car for many days. Cracking a window open brings in road noise and dirt, so maybe you should not smoke in the car at all. One more good reason: you need both hands to drive. Keeping the pipe, cigar, or cigarette in your mouth means running the risk of having hot smoke go directly into your eyes, obscuring road visibility and possibly leading to an accident. As a matter of fact, statistics show that people who smoke while driving have more accidents than nonsmokers.

Smoking is an addiction to nicotine. Stopping is hard but it *can* be done—30 million people have done it already. While it is true that the vast majority of smokers quit on their own, many people do better in organized programs (with and without group support). For more information, contact your local chapter of the American Cancer Society. However, if you must persist in smoking, remember that nonsmokers have rights too!

Mother's Little Helpers—a Modern-Day Fairy Tale

Once upon a time there was a family—Dad, Mom, and three children. Dad had a rewarding job and often came home late in the evening. All three kids were in school. Mom worked part-time, took care of the house and kids and of course Dad. Mom went to work to help "make ends meet." Mom took care of all the carpools, the family laundry and cleaning, the meals, the social calendar, the PTA and school obligations, and relations with the grandparents. Wow, Mom was really something. Look at the things she could do! But Mom began having trouble sleeping, so off she went to her family doctor. She spent exactly 4½ minutes with the kindly doctor, who told her not to worry and gave her a prescription for a sleeping medication. "These will help you to relax," he said as his nurse ushered in the next patient.

Dad said, "I'll help. I will remind you to take your pills." Mom began sleeping better, but pretty soon she felt that she could not sleep if she didn't take the pills. Dad thought the pills must really be working because not only did Mom sleep but she was hot stuff in bed on most nights. Sometimes Mom and Dad had a glass of wine before going to bed. This made Mom a little spacy, but after all she slept well.

One morning Dad had a lot of trouble waking Mom up. He finally succeeded but Mom said she did not feel well. Dad called the friendly doctor. He did not mention the wine they had drunk. The doctor said she should increase the number of Quāaludes she was taking, but only at night before bedtime. That day Mom did not go to work and had lunch with her friend Sally, who knew a lot about life. She told Sally she had been feeling spacy lately and Sally asked her if she was taking any medication. Mom said, "Yes, I'm taking some Quāaludes to help me to sleep." Mom remembered to mention the wine as well. Sally set Mom straight about mixing a hypnotic sedative like Quāaludes with a liquid sedative called alcohol.

That night Mom gave Dad the word: the "little helpers" she needed did not come in a vial of pills. She said, "Dad, I need you and our three children to be my little helpers. I'll sleep just fine if I can have some more help with all the things I have to do around this family." Dad and the kids loved Mom so they all helped out. Mom slept better than ever before. So did Dad and the kids. And they all lived happily (drug-free) ever after.

CHAPTER TWO

Drugs and School

Our children spend the greater part of their waking hours in school. Beyond the nuclear family, the majority of social and emotional learning occurs within and around the school setting. Some of this learning is adventurous and gratifying. Some of it is painful and confusing. All of it determines the quality of the student's life on a daily basis and acts to mold and shape future practices. Since our kids interact socially as well as academically in school, the use of various drugs has implications for both aspects of their lives.

Parents look to the schools to confront and solve the "drug problem." They blame school officials for not stemming the rising tide of drug use. Teachers and school administrators blame parents for failing to properly guide and raise their children. Everyone blames the police for not stopping the seemingly endless flow of drugs available to kids. Overfocusing on the drugs themselves, parents and educators take crash courses in drug terminology and street slang. They are looking through the wrong end of the telescope. We try to scare the kids, con them with pseudoscientific literature, bully them, tail and arrest them and smear them. The kids take the cues and go underground, drugs in tow.

THE EXTENT OF DRUG USE

What you read in the popular press and magazines and see and hear on television and radio may have already convinced you that school-age children are using a wide assortment of drugs. What you have heard is true.

In 1981 the largest study of its kind, involving 17,000 high school seniors from around the nation, was published by the National Institute on Drug Abuse under the title "Highlights from Student Drug Use in America 1975–1980." Tables 1 through 5 on the following pages are taken from this study conducted by Dr. Lloyd Johnson, Dr. Jerald Bachman, and Dr. Patrick O'Malley of the University of Michigan. The information was collected in 1980. Single copies are available at no charge from the National Clearinghouse for Drug Abuse Information (see Appendix C).

At what grade level does the first use of various drugs occur? Table 1 shows the grade of first use for sixteen types of drugs as reported by the senior class of 1980. Initial experimentation with most illicit drugs occurs during the final three years of high school. Each illegal drug, except marijuana, has been used by less than 7 percent of the class by the time they enter tenth grade. However, with marijuana, alcohol, and cigarettes, most of the initial experimentation takes place earlier. For example, daily cigarette smoking was begun by 16 percent prior to tenth grade, followed by only an additional 10 percent after that. The figures for initial use of alcohol are 55 percent prior to and 38 percent following tenth grade; and for marijuana, 31 percent and 29 percent. The "never used" column is quite revealing. By the time they finish their senior year, only 39.7 percent have not tried marijuana, and only 6.8 percent have not tried alcohol.

The age of first use for many of these drugs points to the need for considerable attention to drug prevention programming, both in the home and in the schools, beginning in the middle years of *elementary school.* By the time the kids have reached the junior high school or middle school, experimentation with various drugs has already begun.

Table 2 shows the prevalence and recency of use of eleven

TABLE 1

Grade of First Use for Sixteen Types of Drugs

Grade in Which Drug Was First Used	Marijuana	Inhalants	Amyl/Butyl Nitrites	Hallucinogens	LSD	PCP	Cocaine	Heroin	Other Opiates	Stimulants	Sedatives	Barbiturates	Methaqualone	Tranquilizers	Alcohol	Cigarettes (Daily)
6th	1.9	1.4	0.1	0.1	0.1	0.2	0.1	0.2	0.4	0.3	0.3	0.2	0.1	0.3	8.0	3.0
7–8th	13.0	2.4	1.2	0.8	0.5	1.0	0.5	0.0	0.5	1.5	0.9	0.7	0.3	1.6	22.2	7.2
9th	16.5	1.9	2.2	2.2	1.4	1.9	1.7	0.2	1.8	4.3	2.5	2.3	1.3	3.0	24.8	5.8
10th	14.7	2.5	2.6	3.5	2.2	2.7	3.3	0.2	2.1	6.6	3.3	3.0	1.8	3.3	19.3	4.7
11th	9.7	2.0	3.2	4.3	3.3	2.6	5.8	0.2	3.4	7.3	4.8	3.2	3.3	4.4	11.9	3.4
12th	4.4	1.7	1.8	2.4	1.7	1.0	4.3	0.4	1.6	6.3	3.2	1.6	2.8	2.6	7.0	1.7
Never used	39.7	88.1	88.9	86.7	90.7	90.4	84.3	98.9	90.2	73.6	85.1	89.0	90.5	84.8	6.8	74.2

TABLE 2

Prevalence and Recency of Use
Eleven Types of Drugs

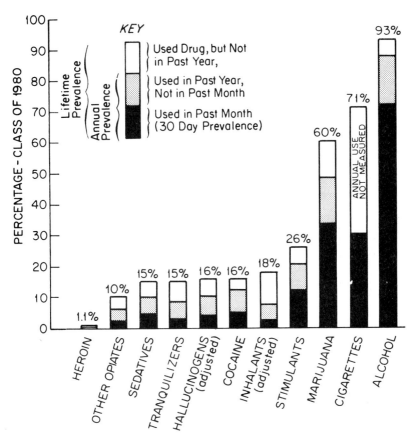

types of drugs as reported by high-school seniors. Before looking at the table, can you guess which drug is the most frequently tried and most regularly and heavily used among youth? If you guessed marijuana or cigarettes you are wrong. Now look at the table.

The answer is *alcohol.* The popularity of this powerful sedative drug warrants equal attention along with all the other drugs of use and potential abuse.

Table 3 shows the trends in annual prevalence of illicit drug use for all seniors who participated in the five years of surveying. In this table, use of "some other illicit drugs" includes any use of hallucinogens, cocaine, and heroin, or any use which is not under a doctor's orders of other opiates, stimulants, sedatives, or tranquilizers.

Table 2 tell us that about two out of every three seniors (65 percent) report illicit drug use at some time in their lives. However, a substantial proportion of them have used only marijuana (28 percent of the sample or 41 percent of all illicit drug users). About four in every ten seniors (39 percent) report using an illicit drug other than marijuana at some time. Marijuana is by far the most widely used illicit drug, with 60 percent reporting some use in their lifetime, 49 percent reporting some use in the past year, and 34 percent use in the past month. The most widely used class of other illicit drugs is stimulants (26 percent lifetime prevalence).

Judging from Table 3, it now appears that 1978 and 1979 may have been the high point in a long and dramatic rise in marijuana use among American high-school students. Until 1978, the proportion of seniors involved in illicit drug use had increased primarily because of the increase in marijuana use. But since 1976 there has been a very gradual, steady increase in the proportion who use some illicit drug other than marijuana, an increase which continued until 1980.

Exposure to drug use by friends is believed to play a pivotal role in initiation into the drug scene. Table 4 shows the proportion of friends using each drug as estimated by seniors in 1980.

If you compare the figures in Table 2 (prevalence and recency of use) and Table 4 (proportion of friends using), you will see how closely personal-use patterns mirror those of friends. The highest levels of exposure involve alcohol and marijuana.

Thirty percent of all seniors say that most or all of their friends get drunk at least once a week! Forty-one percent say they person-

TABLE 3

Trends in Annual Prevalence of Illicit Drug Use, All Seniors

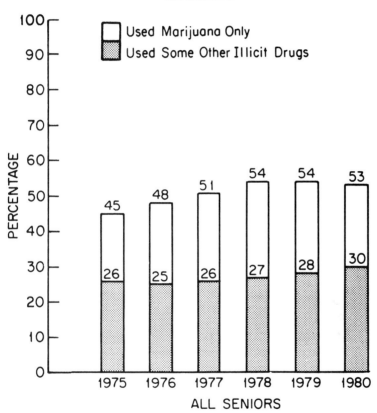

TABLE 4

Proportion of Friends Using Each Drug as Estimated by Seniors in 1980

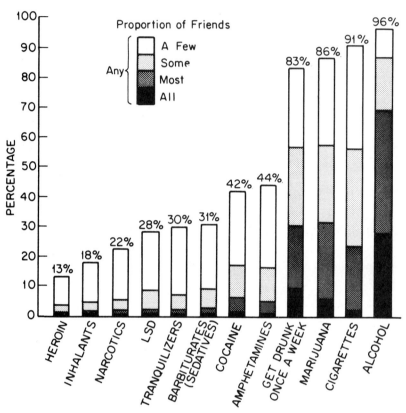

ally had taken five or more drinks in a row during the prior two weeks.

One set of questions in the survey asked for estimates of how difficult it would be to obtain each of a number of different drugs. The answers range across five categories from "probably impossible" to "very easy." Table 5 shows the trends over the five years in perceived availability of drugs.

There are substantial differences in the reported availability of the various drugs. In general, the more widely used drugs

TABLE 5

Trends in Perceived Availability of Drugs

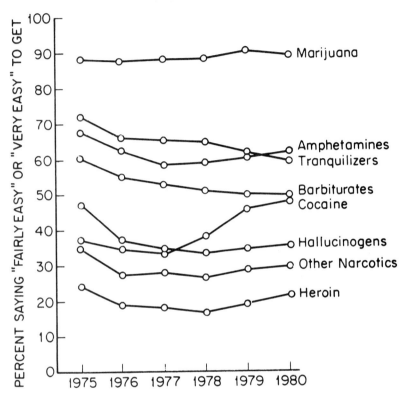

are reported to be the most readily available. Marijuana seems to be almost universally available to high-school seniors; nearly 90 percent report that it would be "very easy" to "fairly easy" for them get it, roughly 30 percent more than the number who report ever having used it. After marijuana, the students indicate that the psychotherapeutic drugs are the most readily available: amphetamines are seen as available by 61 percent, tranquilizers by 59 percent, and barbiturates by 49 percent. Nearly half of the seniors (48 percent) now see cocaine as being available to them.

In 1980 nearly 60 percent of the students said they believed regular marijuana users faced a "great risk" of harming themselves. Three years earlier only 35 percent held that view. In 1978 one in every nine high-school seniors said they were daily users of marijuana. By 1980 the proportion had dropped to one in fourteen. Those who continued to use drugs reported that they now tended to consume smaller amounts and for shorter periods of time. Despite the downward trend, conservative estimates are that, overall, drug use among high-school students remains widespread. Nearly two-thirds of the age group (65 percent) have used an illicit drug, and nearly two out of every five (39 percent) have used an illicit drug other than marijuana. Combined with licit drug use (alcohol, tobacco, etc.), we can see that adolescent drug use is a widespread practice in America.

Just in case you are saying "Thank God my kid only drinks," consider the following information taken from a national study of adolescent drinking behavior involving 5,000 students, age 15 through 17. This study was conducted by the Research Triangle Institute under contract to the National Institute on Alcohol Abuse and Alcoholism and the National Institute on Drug Abuse.[1]

Drinking Levels by Age: 1978 Study

	15	17	18
Abstainer or infrequent	38.6%	29.1%	27.2%
Moderate/heavy or heavier	26.2%	36.3%	36.9%

Moderate/heavy: drank at least once per week with 2 to 4 drinks per occasion, or drank 3 to 4 times per month having more than 5 drinks at a time.
Heavier: drank once a week and had at least 5 drinks per occasion.

1. "Heavier" drinker characterized almost 15 percent of the tenth- to twelfth-graders; 17.3 percent were "moderate/heavy" drinkers; and more than one in four drank at least once a week.

2. By the tenth grade, about seven out of ten students could no longer be called "abstainers." The data show

that three out of five kids drank at least once per month. (There are more than 11 million tenth- to twelfth-graders in America.)

3. Three out of ten teenagers in the tenth to twelfth grades could be considered problem drinkers: he or she was drunk at least six times within a year, or experienced negative consequences of drinking two or more times in at least three of six life areas (friends, family, school, dates, police, driving).

4. About one in four reported having driven after having a good bit to drink, and one out of ten reported having done this at least four times within the past year. Car accidents are a leading cause of death among sixteen- to nineteen-year-olds.

5. Comparison data show that the gap between boys and girls is closing. In 1974, 18 percent more girls than boys were moderate drinkers or less. By 1978 this gap had closed to 13 percent. And 19 percent more boys than girls fell into the higher drinking categories in 1974, but in 1978 the difference was just 14 percent.

Young people who drink heavily tend to do less well in school than those who don't drink as much. They also tend to smoke marijuana more and are involved in "unconventional" behavior. While personality and environmental influences are seen as underlying causes, it is reasonable to assert that for teenagers who drink, the chances they will engage in other problem behaviors are greater than for those who don't drink.

College-bound youth report less drug use than those students who are not college bound. Neither of the studies just cited addresses a newer and possibly more dangerous set of practices, namely that of multiple substance use and abuse. Many young people report drug combinations, marijuana and alcohol being the most popular of the mixtures.

A large proportion of youths who become involved in illicit drug use also become multiple drug users. Listed below are the number of additional drugs regularly used by the habitual users

Multiple Drug Use[2]

of those who reported regularly* using:	number of clients	% of the sample	have, on the average, also regularly used the following number of other drugs
marijuana	2,363	86%	3.2
alcohol	2,196	80	3.4
inhalants	525	19	4.5
other drugs	28	1	4.7
amphetamines	890	32	5.3
heroin	215	8	5.4
hashish	754	27	5.5
barbiturates	811	29	5.5
tranquilizers	581	21	5.8
hallucinogens	656	24	5.8
PCP (Phencyclidine)	611	22	5.8
cocaine	263	10	6.0
over-the-counter drugs	136	5	6.2
illegal methadone	49	2	6.2
other opiates	397	14	6.3

* Regular use is defined as weekly or greater use for a period of at least one month.

for each of several drug categories. These figures represent youths twelve to nineteen years of age who were admitted to treatment for drug abuse.

Overwhelming evidence from numerous studies has documented the widespread use of many drugs on college campuses throughout America. You need only to amplify the findings regarding high-school drug use to get some idea of the extent of use in college. College has always served as the setting in which many young people are introduced to alcohol, and many fraternities pride themselves on the ability of their members to put away voluminous amounts of the stuff. A 1982 study[3] of college deans at 181 two-year and four-year colleges and universities in the U.S. found that about 75 percent of students are drinkers. The same study showed that one of six college students drinks excessively and more than one of fifty must leave school ultimately because of drinking problems. The deans classified about half the students as social or experimental drinkers but said 16 percent drank excessively. Colleges have become alarmed at the large amount of drinking on campus and consequent vandalism (as much as 80 percent may be alcohol related). And in traffic accident deaths, half of the 13,370 deaths of people aged eighteen to twenty-four in 1981 were alcohol related. The general perception held by faculty and students is that drinking cannot be stopped, so more and more schools are trying to encourage moderation and responsible drinking behavior. Colleges are employing many measures toward this goal: weekend pickup services for students too drunk to drive, alcohol awareness classes, encouraging drinking within walking distance of living areas (some schools have bars right on campus), student-to-student breathylizer tests to keep blood alcohol levels within legal limits, serving of nonalcoholic beverages at parties. Age limits are being raised for alcohol use. New Jersey, New York, and Connecticut are just a few states that have recently raised the legal drinking age. Students are bitter, claiming that if they are old enough to fight for their country and vote, they are old enough to drink. Most don't believe that changing the laws will actually lower the incidence of young adult drinking. As one college freshman pointed out, "There's plenty of phony identification papers for sale and you can always get a senior to buy booze for you. Bartenders may laugh at phony papers but they will serve you anyway."

Drugs have joined alcohol on the college campus, leading to new patterns of multiple substance use. Parents have wondered what factors tend to place their children at risk before and during the college years. One study,[4] which focused on religiosity and drug use, helped to identify historical (precollege) and current characteristics of high-risk undergraduates.

The study further shows that among frequent users, Jewish students were more likely to be involved in multiple use of drugs other than alcohol; non-Jewish students were more inclined to report heavy use of alcoholic beverages. "Traditionally, Jews have

Drug Abuse Risk Factors for College Students

Past-History Factors	Current Risk Factors
1. History of regular cigarette smoking	1. Poor academic performance
2. History of trouble with the law	2. Dissatisfaction with school
3. Lack of close relationships with parents	3. Widespread peer-group drug usage
4. Never attended religious services	4. No current religious preference
	5. Lack of a strong sense of purpose in life
	6. Tendency to minimize the importance of material accomplishments and to emphasize the importance of values such as freedom and equality

placed great emphasis on academic and professional achievement. It is therefore not surprising to find that, among Jewish students, underachievers in school and those who perceived their college studies to be unrelated to career and life goals were likely to be frequent drug users." The study helps us to see how movement away from traditional values—a history of not attending religious services or no current religious preference—is often associated with drug use. Other studies point to the fact that when young adults escalate their drug use beyond alcohol and marijuana, their academic performance tends to go down.

Drug-use trends are rarely static in nature. They have a way of changing in terms of drug popularity, drug combinations, amount of use, and frequency of use. Let's trace the natural history of one contemporary drug to make this point. Acid (LSD) was first synthesized in 1938, but its hallucinogenic effects were not discovered until 1943 when Dr. Albert Hoffman accidentally ingested some of the drug and recorded the first acid trip. Drs. Timothy Leary and Richard Alpert began studies of the drug in the early 1960s at Harvard's Center for Research in Personality. Students in the Cambridge area began "turning on and tuning in" to the psychedelic (mind-expanding) effects of LSD. The Harvard establishment put the kibosh on student tripping and the experimenters moved their research efforts to the International Federation for Internal Freedom (IFIF) at Cambridge and Zihuatanejo, Mexico. The media picked up on the early reports of acid's ability to induce powerful hallucinations and to tickle and enhance sexual fancies; it became the new drug of rebellion. Between 1963 and 1965 the scientific and popular accounts of the drug stressed pleasure and exploration of consciousness. As a consequence the drug's popularity grew, especially on college campuses. It was not until 1967 that reports of abuse, bad trips, and flashbacks led to the drug's first bad press—again initially in scientific papers and then in the popular media. Use began to wane by the early 1970s and with it the "death" of the peace and love movement. New times demanded new drugs and the search for the safe mind-altering drug continues unabated. Acid seems to be making a comeback, particularly on the west coast, as earlier reports of chromosome damage remain unproven. While acid use flowed and then ebbed, a sister psychedelic drug (albeit far less potent) continued to grow and has virtually been institutionalized in the America drug scene—namely marijuana.

One of the raging controversies of the drug scene for many years has been the "stepping stone" theory that experimentation with and use of one drug can lead to curiosity about other drugs. Some studies point to an association between the use of one substance and future use of other substances. However, there is no evidence that once you use one drug you are locked into a pattern of automatically escalating drug abuse. We have already mentioned some risk factors which seem to predispose young people to drug use and/or abuse. However, as no evidence has established the existence of an "addictive" personality, we must understand that the issue is far more complicated than some of the antidrug forces would have us believe. Certain practical associations do exist. For example, it is known that people who smoke cigarettes are more likely to try marijuana, which is commonly smoked (but can also be eaten). Influences to try alcohol and marijuana usually come from best friends. But the risk factors that can lead to other drug use and abuse are combinations of peer and parental influence, age of first use (the younger you are when you start, the greater the chances of future problems), quality of adolescent/parent relationships, the behavioral model parents provide, parental expectations, and the degree to which deviance is tolerated in the household. It isn't as simple as some would have us believe, i.e., if you smoke pot you will become a heroin addict! Nonsense, despite the fact that most heroin addicts have smoked pot. Again, the relationships as determined by careful study show that there are many overlapping causes of drug use and drug abuse.

There has been a lot of alarm recently about adolescent drinking. We must learn to pay close attention to the terminology employed to describe the use of alcohol. The media often speak about teenage "alcoholism" in their attempts to try to sell newspapers or TV advertising time. Television news coverage focuses primarily on tragedy and gossip. The more sensational, the better. However, the actual number of teenage alcoholics is not known, and while a serious problem for these young people and their families, it is not the pattern of alcohol use that most of us need fear in our young. Alcoholism is out-of-control drinking; it is an inability to use alcohol the way most other people do. The alcoholic usually cannot predict in any episode of drinking how much he or she will consume or what the effects will be. Most adolescent drinkers do not fit this description. Our primary concern must be with the dangers associated with a single episode of drinking in which judgment is impaired. One need not be an "alcoholic" to get into a fight, become pregnant, wreck a car, or commit vandalism. Fifty-five percent of alcohol experimentation occurs before entrance into high school. Helping our kids to deal with this reality and all that it may imply at such a young age is the greater task.

The drug problem is not a drug problem as much as it is a people problem. Therefore, alcohol-specific programs of prevention are probably worthless. It is common to find other problems in the lives of young people with drinking problems (other drug use, family discord, deviant behavior), and a more general syndrome of behavior requires something more than an understanding of a specific chemical or drug. Problem drinkers don't live the same kinds of lives as social drinkers. More is at issue than the alcohol. We must work with issues such as family life, self-image, multiple substance abuse, social acceptance, and adolescent sexuality. There are ways that we can help:

- Recognize that young people and adults use drugs for certain reasons and be open to a discussion of the reasons without lecturing.

- At least half the young lie to their parents about illicit drug use (such as marijuana). They do so because they fear punishment and don't want their parents to think badly of them. We must respect forthrightness in our young people but also understand their need for privacy.

- Keep channels of communication open. Drugs, sex, rejection, body image—these are difficult things to discuss, especially with parents. We must encourage kids to state their feelings and ideas even when they differ radically from our own.

- Adults have the right and responsibility to state their opinions and feelings as well. Young people need us to be there for them with our knowledge and experience. They don't appreciate wishy-washy adults. At least agree to disagree.

- Adults should get active in school boards and parents' associations. Make sure your children's schools are addressing social and emotional needs, not just intellectual needs. Make sure school-based drug programs are focusing on the context and issues within the life of adolescents and not just on the pharmacology of drugs.

- When dealing with a young person with a drinking prob-

lem, be on the alert for parental alcohol abuse or alcoholism (if one parent is an alcoholic there is a one-in-four
chance of the offspring being alcoholic; if both parents
are alcoholics there is a one-in-two chance).
- Many kids get high (on various drugs) because they can't
handle their own emerging sexuality. Provide them with
factual information and emotional support about human
sexuality.

DRUGS AND STUDYING

Over the generations students have learned to use a variety
of drugs, both licit and illicit, as study aids. Much of this activity
is associated with periods of intensive studying usually referred
to as "cramming." Although most students, including those who
keep up with the work all semester long, tend to cram just before
exams, many are trying to play catch-up in a very risky way.
The drugs people use to stay awake during cramming can have
some bad side effects and aftereffects. We live in an "instant"
society. We want everything to happen fast and easy. Here are
several vignettes which show how things can go wrong.

When I was working nights as a nursing student, I could
never get used to sleeping during the day. I guess my biological clocks did not want to change. So I started taking amphetamines [very powerful stimulants]. I used the spansules.
Throughout the night I would be given to sudden bursts
of frenetic energy during which time I was racing up and
down the hallways. When the night shift ended I was so
wired I had to take some barbiturates [sedatives] to calm
me down enough to fall asleep. I got off that roller coaster
after just one week.

Back when I was a freshman in college I took an urban
planning course. There was no midterm and we had to ab-
sorb a lot of material for the final exam. Jeff had been taking
incredible amounts of No-Doz [primary ingredient is caf-

feine, a stimulant] and drinking pots of coffee [more caffeine]. He stayed up for forty-eight hours straight, studying. On the day of the final he sat in front of me. Five minutes into the exam he fell asleep. I tried to wake him. I poked him in the ribs, pinched him, talked right into his ear— nothing worked. It was very weird. As soon as the exam ended he woke up, staggered back to his room, and slept for twenty-three hours. He flunked the course.

Sheila was really uptight about the big examination in chemistry. She had found that smoking grass relaxed her at other times. So she figured right before the test should help. She got relaxed all right. She was so blissed out that she found the chemistry formulas and equations floating around in one big sea of symbols and numbers in her head. She knew the stuff but could not seem to concentrate and put it all together. She also kept losing track of time. She should have gotten at least a B but ended up with a low C.

By the time I reached my junior year of college I had been drinking pretty steadily. At first I just drank at parties on weekends but I started to party during the week as well. There was always an ample supply of grass and booze in the dorm. My grades stayed up so I did not think I had a problem. It got to the point where I was drinking daily. At the end of the fall semester I studied real hard to prepare for finals. When I sat down to take my math final I ended up staring at a blank page for two hours. I knew I knew the material but could simply not recall any of it. I later learned that I had been having blackouts, which are periods in which short-term memory is disrupted by alcohol.

While it is true that stimulant drugs will keep you awake, they have sometimes been known to play nasty tricks with memory circuits. They do provide a sense of energy but also make it difficult not to fidget, and one can become distracted easily. Time perceptions may be slightly altered and feelings of fear can be intensified. Symptoms of caffeinism closely mirror those of an anxiety condition (see Chapter 3 for details), some of which can hamper rather than enhance test-taking ability. Tranquilizers, on the other hand, can remove that competitive edge. A little test anxiety seems to improve test performance. Too much test anxiety can overwhelm us. If we take drugs in addition to being anxious about the material to be absorbed, the results can be disastrous. Drugs that speed up or slow down the electrochemical processes involved in memory and concentration can be risky. People have walked out of exams feeling, in their drug-induced state, that they had done marvelously well, only to discover they had failed miserably. There is a thin line between the advantage to be gained and the edge to be lost when using drugs to aid in studying and exam taking. Proper study regimens and good health are far more helpful than the unpredictable interactions between the stress of exams and the physical and mental effects of the drugs. The whole idea of waiting until the last moment to study almost guarantees this volatile combination of events.

It is becoming a real goof for more and more kids to go to school high on either grass or alcohol. Kids like to get a big kick out of fooling their teachers. They brag about how naive their teachers are and how hip they are. Most kids believe that alcohol can interfere with schoolwork more than grass can. Common reasons for getting high before class are wanting to feel relaxed, getting through a boring class, and imitating friends. Interestingly, some students can learn while high, while others get too confused or disoriented to do so. It's a risky business at best, and doesn't really make a boring lecture any more interesting. There is always the chance of being caught by school officials, having one's parents brought in, and being suspended. Any student who uses drugs too often, specifically drugs which inhibit memory function and concentration, can end up with poor grades even if everything else in his or her life is okay.

It is not easy to sit down and discuss drugs with your kids. One major study showed that 55 percent of parents never discuss drugs with their children. Clearly the time has come for all parents to face the issue squarely. Here are some questions that can guide you into a frank discussion of the relationship between your youngster's drug and study habits. These questions can be presented in a rhetorical fashion to let your kids know you care. They don't necessarily have to answer them in front of you. It may be better to let them give oblique responses. They'll get the message that you have legitimate concerns without your accusing them of having done anything wrong.

- Have they ever noticed that their grades have suffered when using drugs?
- Have they ever gone to school high?
- Have they ever had trouble concentrating on schoolwork when using drugs?
- Do they get high and party when they should be studying?
- Do they use drugs to help them study?
- Have their teachers ever expressed concern to them about drug use?
- Do all of their friends use drugs?
- Do they cut class to get high?
- Are they using lunch money to buy drugs?
- Is cramming their only method of studying?

These questions are loaded! Again, your child does not have to answer them directly. They are really just a listing of important concerns for both child and adult. The challenge to any student is to seek a balance between studies and pleasure. Those students who value education will find a way not to allow partying to interfere with the work of learning. Most young people I have known who do well in school and also use drugs for recreational purposes (only) have applied the following practices:

1. Drugs do not play a central role in their lives.
2. They are knowledgeable about the drugs they use and are very careful about their drug sources.
3. They never traffic in drugs; they get drugs only from close friends.
4. They don't use drugs as study aids. They watch their health around exam time.

77

5. They don't care what kids deeper into the drug culture think of them.

6. When they use drugs they do so in moderation.

7. They study hard all week, reserving the weekends for partying.

The unmotivated or failing student is most at risk for drug use and abuse. As parents, we must stay on top of our children's school performance so that we may assist them if they get into academic difficulties. To fail to do so increases the risks of drug abuse and makes communication increasingly difficult.

PEER-GROUP PRESSURE

There is an important relationship between peer-group pressure and drug use. Although peer pressure is widely thought to be an issue primarily with young people, the pressure on adults is just as strong. Of course, no one factor can totally account for a person's becoming involved with drugs. There is almost always more than one reason:

1. Drugs make me feel good—I like to get high.

2. Self-medication against feelings of tension, anxiety, and depression.

3. The individual's attitude toward society and the "establishment."

4. Poor family relationships.

5. Boredom.

6. Parental drug-taking behavior.

7. A search for altered states of consciousness.

8. Age: the earlier one is exposed to drug experimentation, the greater the likelihood of continued experimentation and use.

9. Lack of religious affiliation (religiosity).

10. Availability of drugs.

11. Lack of interest in academic life.
12. Absence of goal orientation.
13. Disregard of the law (illicit drugs).

Several of these factors can interrelate and have at least some bearing on peer relations. For young people drugs and alcohol have become an integral part of the youth scene. Their social and cultural world interacts with the larger society in which drugs have become common. Movie plots, television programs, rock and folk music, tee shirts, jewelry—all reflect the drug aspects of the youth and adult cultures. Using drugs as an adolescent is a rite of passage into adulthood. It is a way to grow up, be hip, and leave childhood and parental control behind. Drugs such as alcohol and marijuana have been "institutionalized" as part of the youth scene.

Peer relations start with a single friend, not with the large group. In one study of marijuana and other drug use, it was found that marijuana use by a best friend was the factor which correlated most strongly with the probability and frequency of marijuana use among high-school students, outranking personal, family, or sociodemographic factors. When the study looked at drug use beyond marijuana to other illicit drugs, however, parental and personal attributes were found to increase while peer influences decreased in importance. For these young people, factors such as depression, school performance, educational aspirations, closeness to parents, and reported parental drug use were more important than peer influences.

Experimentation with marijuana and alcohol depends strongly on what close friends and the broader peer group are into. Kids who get into heavier drug usage become members of other and ever-dwindling circles of kids, who usually have drug and nondrug problems coming down on them. This is certainly true of young people and adults who use drugs habitually and compulsively. It is a fact of adolescent life that kids who use drugs and alcohol have more friends who also use drugs and alcohol than "straight" friends. This excerpt of a conversation among a group of tenth-graders (sophomore year of high school, age fifteen) makes the point very clearly.

> JOHN: Most kids have tried booze or grass. I only know a few who haven't.
>
> BETH: I think it depends on who your friends are. I would never have dreamed of smoking dope if my two best friends weren't doing it.
>
> PEGGY: You know those kids who hang around the mall near the rear parking lot? They're into some heavy drugs. I don't even see them at school anymore.
>
> JOHN: Yeah, Charlie ——— hangs out with them. He's really messed up. I heard he got caught trying to sell some pills to an eighth-grader.
>
> SUSAN: Most kids don't get into that scene. You know, they just party a little on the weekends. Like us.
>
> PEGGY: That's true, Susan. You can't do drugs during the week and expect to handle all that homework.

In many ways, this conversation typifies the drug experience for most kids. They accept drugs (including alcohol) as part of their world, they speak nonchalantly about them (most of the time), they see real differences between occasional use and regular use, they don't let drugs interfere with other activities (like school or athletics), and they either look down on or worry about kids who are into heavy drug use.

However, what if other kids' opinions and other factors have led your child into this smaller circle of regular drug users? Then everything is inverted. Drugs are a central part of life, kids who don't do what they are doing are "square" or "out of it," sports and academic success are downplayed or ridiculed, and so on. Either way the social milieu is a powerful factor.

Dealing and coping with peer-group pressure can be a difficult experience for all of us. However, with the increasing emphasis on assertiveness in American life, some valuable lessons can be taken from that experience. For most of us it comes down to not saying yes when we really want to say no. Here are some thoughts that may help you and your kids work out your own attitudes toward that very real pressure when it comes along—and it will.

1. Realize that your children will be subjected to these pressures from time to time and that they will have important decisions to make. Help them to understand that these are their own decisions, and that they, not their friends, are the ones who will have to live with the consequences.

2. Explain to them that good, caring friends will want to share experiences with them that they regard as positive (this includes getting high). Also explain that good friends may enthusiastically suggest, but will not ram it down their throats or deride them when they say no. A good friend may try to talk them into it but won't really dump on them for continuing to refuse. Anyone who does is no friend.

3. Tell your kids that from time to time they will not wish to do something they may have done previously with friends. "I'm not in the mood" is all they should have to say. If their friends come down on them, it's the friends' problem, not their own.

4. Help them to understand that many times we begin acting and dressing a certain way because we wish to be accepted by a certain group. Help them to ask themselves if belonging to a group by adopting the group's "image" is what they are after, or do they want genuine friendship with members of that group?

5. Tell them to be prepared to get their feelings hurt. Saying no can lead to rejection. There is no way to avoid hurt feelings if they are going to become their own person. But these feelings will pass a lot quicker than the guilt of going against their own values (selling out).

6. Advise them to keep in mind that, when they do use drugs, they don't have to simply mimic the other kids.

Encourage them to get to know their own limits and to stick with them. Let the next person show off. How much is not the same as how good.

7. Sometimes a white lie can get your child out of the pressure cooker. One of my favorites is "The doctor has me on medication and I can't mix it with anything else," or try "I'm into abstinence this month." The idea is not to say yes when you really want to say no.

8. Encourage them not to fear saying "Let me think about that for a while." After all, it's their health, physical and mental, that is at stake.

9. Ask them to take a hard look at the group of kids they wish to identify with. If using drugs is the only way in, then they ought to think long and hard about why that is. The group may be more interested in conformity to their norms than in your child as an individual. Tell your children to check out other groups who will accept them for what they are already and not what the group wants them to become.

CLIQUES AND POPULARITY

Adolescence is a time when kids actively try on various identities in their search for their own. "Who am I?" is a vital question some people spend a lifetime pursuing. It becomes a particularly acute question in the middle-school and high-school years.

We, as adults, often accuse young people of being conformists when they are usually only playing a game we invented. In their school years, kids tend to separate into various cliques. It is still the exceptional child who is a loner. These cliques go under various names in different parts of the country. Here are a few:

Hitters: used to be called "rocks" in my old neighborhood. These are the tough kids. They are into physical power. They get their kicks by bullying and intimidating other kids. Often called "rowdies" by other kids.

Eggheads: sometimes called "squares." These are the kids who excel academically in school. They are college-bound and serious about their studies. They evoke a lot of envy on the part of other kids.

Heads: These are the kids who are really into drugs. They are often blatant in their drug use. Their lives seem to center around anything to do with drugs and getting high.

Jocks: In any neck of the woods these are the kids who are into athletics and varsity sports. They are often into body building as well.

Lovers: These are the kids who really get into dating and relationships. They never seem to be without a partner but change them quite often. Usually hang around with other kids who are into their scene.

Rockers: not to be confused with hitters. These kids are into rock music and styles in a big way. Most recently they are into "punk" and "new wave." You can catch some strange hair colors in this group.

Goody-Goodies: Harder to stereotype. Usually refers to school leaders, religious kids, school club members, and those perceived as "teacher's pets."

What images do these stereotypes conjure up in your own mind? The mere fact that you can probably elaborate on any one of these shows how powerful they are. Kids want desperately to belong to one or more of these groups. They often go from one to the other, seeing where they can make friends, be accepted, and get comfortable. Sometimes the groups overlap.

Which of these groups use drugs? To some extent they all do. At least they tend to experiment. Some of them, like the heads, the rockers, and the hitters, are better known for their prominent use of drugs. Have you ever heard stories about how much beer the jocks can consume or the steroids they sometimes take or the amphetamines that get them up for the big game? How about the wide assortment of drugs that the lovers prefer (cocaine, marijuana, Quāaludes, amyl and butyl nitrates)? And of course everybody likes to drink. You see the point. All kinds of kids use drugs for all kinds of reasons.

All groups develop norms over time, that is, a common set of beliefs and behaviors. It is important to know the norms of the different cliques. Your kid will have to measure his or her own emerging values against those of the group. But loneliness and a strong desire to belong are powerful motives. So kids join various cliques to get a sense of relatedness and to get into the social scene. As parents you should know who your kids' friends are, where and how they spend their time, and such things as when they are coming home. You can make your feelings known about the people they associate with, but then stand back and allow them to sort things out on their own. Sometimes strongly objecting to their friends guarantees that they will spend more time with them. You must discuss with your kids where to draw the line (for example, establish that you don't want them hanging around with kids who are experimenting with hard drugs or getting into vandalism). Again, short of forbidding certain associations, you must allow them to experiment with new social connections, making and breaking them as *they* see fit. The best you can hope for is that they will seek out your advice and bounce their feelings off you.

Many parents allow themselves to believe that kids who use drugs don't go out for athletics. It's true that the kids who end up in drug treatment programs usually shy away from academic and athletic competition. But this has led to the creation of a myth, that athletes don't use drugs. You have just read about the major ways in which sports and drugs have mixed. If your youngsters wish to enter into competitive athletics (no matter what sport—don't think golfers or tennis players don't get high), then be sure you and the kids do so with your eyes wide open. Here are some guidelines to help keep sports and drugs separate and not equal.

- Find out the coach's policies and attitudes regarding the use of drugs. Some coaches take a very hard line about party drugs and sports, and kids have been kicked off teams for breaking the rules.
- Find out if the team has a "play at all costs—win at all costs" mentality. This is where kids tend to misuse painkillers, whether prescribed by team physicians or family doctors. Misuse of painkillers can lead to a "medical addiction." Remember, pain is a symptom; the underlying cause should be diagnosed (through examination and x-ray procedures). "Toughing it out" can lead to permanent physical disabilities.
- State your position about the use of stimulants. Let your son or daughter know that they have to make it with natural ability. Drugs can ruin concentration and only make athletes "feel" more powerful. They don't actually create power or strength.
- High-school athletes who celebrate after the big game often drive cars. Drugging, drinking, and driving don't mix. A local athlete in my community had a full football scholarship nipped in the bud when he mixed booze, pills, and fast driving. His kidney was punctured in the resulting crash.
- Another risk to budding young athletes' dreams of college scholarships is getting busted for possessing or selling drugs. Colleges don't draft ball players with criminal records.
- There are no chemical shortcuts to hard workouts, proper diet, healthful sleep, and a keen mental edge.

Kids and adults often tell us that getting high can be a pleasant experience, bringing people closer together. Chemicals can break the ice and help us to get rid of some of our social inhibitions, but I do not believe that drugs help people get closer. Drugs can make you "feel" closer, but a close relationship, whether it's between lovers, friends, or relatives, requires hard work. The transient bliss that drugs can produce is no substitute for hard-won affection and respect. Relationships are supposed to have ups and downs. If you or your kids are using drugs to smooth out the rough spots, then you are only deluding yourselves. You may find, in time, that the rough spots can become the reason for losing someone, because you used drugs to ignore them. Here are some pointers that can help your family understand whether your social relationships are being helped or hurt by drugs. The questions are reflective, that is, they are designed to help you ask yourselves some tough questions as a family. Adults can start by volunteering information about themselves.

1. Do you and your friends always get high when you are together?
2. Do drugs seem to dominate the conversations?
3. Do your friends give you grief if you choose not to join them in using drugs?
4. Do you ever get the feeling (in relationships with the opposite sex) that your partner needs to get high in order to enjoy being with you?
5. Does everything you do with your friends have to be experienced through drugs (music, sex, movies, rapping, dancing)?
6. Do your friends keep telling you, in so many words, that their motto in life is "Better living through chemistry"?
7. Do you really know your friends as people? Do they know you?
8. Are your social relationships better when you are high?

If you are unhappy with your answers to these questions, then it is time for you to take a hard look at how you are relating to the friends in your life. If drugs seem to be central to these relationships, maybe you got stoned and missed the intimacy of real friendship. Life is a study in contrasts. People who never try drugs may be missing something, but people who use drugs a lot are usually hiding from others and/or themselves.

SCHOOL-BASED PREVENTION PROGRAMS

Parents too often leave it entirely up to the schools to educate their children about drugs. Chapter 1 has suggested some specific ways of addressing this issue in your own family. Your interest in educating young people should not stop within the confines of your own family. Parents have a strong and positive role to play in supporting and aiding school-based prevention programs. This can be accomplished by being active on school boards and parents associations, and by playing a direct role in the school drug prevention program by speaking with other parents and assisting staff and students.

Administrative support: Everything flows from the top in bureaucracies like schools. Therefore it is essential that the top administrators of your kids' school back the program from its very inception. They control the important logistical supports which are needed for a good program: space allocation; released time for teachers and students for training and program operation/participation; budget for educational materials; communications with students, teachers, and parents. Administrators need to hear from parents. So let them know that you demand quality prevention programs for your kids.

Faculty support: In most schools today teachers are fairly well aware of the impact of drug use and abuse on the student body and on themselves as educators. They will usually give tacit approval to any reasonable approach and more explicit support for programs that they can believe in (based on sound educational principles). Parents should not be alarmed when only a handful of teachers volunteer for prevention programs. You want to involve only those teachers who are really motivated. Ask the kids; they will tell you which teachers they can talk to and really respect.

Parental support: Often the most neglected and yet the most concerned group in the school universe, parents must become directly involved in school prevention programming. You need to know that your kids' school is doing something in the area of drug abuse prevention. Parents should be involved from the earliest stages of such programs. Even if you are not clear as to what roles can be played by parents, you can promote the program through the school board, parents' associations, and meetings with school administrators. Confidentiality issues may prevent parents from getting involved in counseling aspects of your school's program. However, there are many things you can do such as organizing and leading parent discussion groups, reaching out to parents of kids in trouble, clerical support, trips, dramatics, help with phone work, and so on.

Drug education materials: All materials should be scientifically accurate and free of the half-truths, emotional biases, and scare tactics that have, in the past, caused young people to reject them out of hand. I have never been able to compete (in the public-relations sense) with the law-enforcement officers on the panels on which I have served. They come armed with suitcases filled with drugs and drug paraphernalia and horror stories of addiction, overdose, and painful withdrawal. This "bread and circuses" approach always pulls the adults and kids away from considering issues of personal responsibility to ogling gaudy displays of homemade hypodermic needles, hash pipes, glassine envelopes (filled with adulterated heroin), and marijuana joints. Fortunately the police always stop short of showing the audience how to cook and shoot up the dope. A screening committee of students, teachers, and parents can review all proposed books, tapes, films, pamphlets, and speakers before allowing their general distribution.

Role of students: It is a real pitfall to conceive of the students solely in the role of passive recipients of such programs. In order to work, the program must actively belong to them. The programs most acceptable to the student body are those which are student-run and faculty-advised. The greater the role of a select group of well-motivated students in the planning and running of the program, the greater the chances of general student acceptance. The kids who do well in such program involvement:

1. are doing well in school,
2. are liked by other kids,
3. want to work with (not "treat") other kids,
4. have nonrigid attitudes about drug use but generally aren't into drugs, and
5. are plugged into nonchemical ways of having fun.

Kids who used to do drugs should not be excluded if they meet the other criteria. Students are your best bet for creating counter-peer-group pressure. Kids in trouble with drugs don't have non-drug-using friends. The students running your school program can reach out to them, providing new circles of "straight" friends.

The planning committee: This should be composed of faculty, students, administrators, and parents. At the beginning, everyone should feel free to brainstorm. This will help to set the goals for the program. Be realistic here, as change is difficult and success feeds upon itself. Setting modest aims and getting people used to the idea of a new program is enough of a task to keep you all busy for a while.

One of the most difficult and important decisions you will have to make is how to spell out the nature of the program. Will it be identified as and limited to issues of drug use? Or will it have a broader context, dealing with issues concerning all school-age kids, drugs being only one among them? In middle- and high-school settings, when you give the program a drug identity you almost always ensure its failure. This is where you must work out your program philosophy. If you think the drug problem is simply limited to the drugs themselves, then you will miss the single most important lesson of the last two decades: drugs are a people issue! When seeking to mount a program you must create a context in which the many causes of drug experimentation, use, abuse, and addiction are considered. Drug-information-only programs have proven to be ineffective, incomplete, possibly even dangerous, and have generally failed to have the needed impact of a genuinely preventive program. Listen to one of our teachers after two years of involvement:

> When we started out I thought this was going to be an easy job. All I would have to do is memorize all the drug names and effects and warn kids about the dangers. After my first lecture to the kids I found out that they knew more than I did anyway. So I had to realize that the kids had as many and often the same reasons for using drugs as adults I know had for drinking alcohol. From that point on I stopped focusing on the drugs and started trying to get to know the kids. This is when the whole thing came alive for me. I got closer to the kids, started listening more and talking less, and together we struggled toward a prevention program.

Curriculum: There are any number of published curricula which one can learn about by contacting your state drug authority and the National Institute on Drug Abuse (NIDA). You must make sure that the outlined approach will meet the needs of your school. The best curricula are those which are graduated by students' ages. The curriculum must be dynamic, not static. Curricula are only guidelines, not a rehash of the Ten Commandments. There must be a built-in give-and-take. Kids are tired of lectures. Affective education, values clarification, rap groups, habit management—these are the ways to bring across the material. Kids pick up on these formats and really get into them. The only approaches which rigorous research has been able to support in primary prevention are these "new generation" strategies: affective, peer-oriented, and multidimensional approaches.

Physical setting: The program can be run in any number of settings. It is a good idea to set aside a particular schoolroom as a "rap room." This is the kind of place that students can decorate according to their own tastes and feel comfortable in.

The room has to ensure privacy and should be away from the main flow of traffic.

Confidentiality: This can be a tricky business. On the one hand you want the kids who are abusing drugs to come to the program, but you are afraid that they won't if the program can't ensure their anonymity. In many states, children are the property (chattel) of their parents, and the parents have a right to know what is happening. Drugs do kill and harm people. The program must abide by various federal, state, and local laws. A general rule of thumb is that the kid must be able to come to the program in confidence. Once he or she has revealed a personal drug problem, the staff must make a determination. If the student can get it together (stop abusing drugs) by joining a program, fine. But if the student is out of control, then the program administrators have a moral (if not legal) obligation to inform the child's family. Parents should lobby for this, and school programs should be "neutral" territory. This is a program policy issue that must be worked out very carefully. There is no room for confusion when people's well-being and the long arm of the law are involved. Some kids are really afraid of terrible consequences at home if their folks find out they are using drugs. Programs must help them to understand that they only contribute to their continued drug abuse by keeping it a secret. The time has come for us to consider a family component to our school prevention programs. When dealing with drug abusers I have found it very useful to introduce the child's parents to other parents I know who have lived through the same experience.

Integrated approach: Schools should be just as interested in issues such as adolescent social and emotional growth and health as they are in academic performance. We should all be upset by the fact that most school administrators take for granted that these issues are addressed in traditional educational approaches. At best, they are by-products of a sound curriculum; at worst, they are totally ignored. We like to talk about preparing the students for the "real" world they will face after graduation.

What about the reality of their daily lives, in and out of school? Schools are wonderful places for kids to learn about the changes their bodies are going through, the realities of competition and cooperation, conformity behavior, responsibility for one's self, human psychology, family dynamics, and so much more. Should these things be taught instead of the three R's? Of course not! These issues should be the context in which the fundamentals are taught. And they all tie in to our concern here: the kids' ability to deal with the drug culture in a responsible way.

Prevention of what? If the major goal of drug prevention programs to date has been primary prevention—stopping young people from experimenting with drugs—we have failed miserably. It may even be that by paying so much attention to the informational approach and letting media hype serve as our main vehicle, we have created the very monster we thought we were slaying. For example, made-for-television movies and docudramas seem to deal only with the horrors of teenage addiction or alcoholism. Think about this the next time you see a TV movie about a twelve-year-old girl, strung out on dope and selling her body. What did you learn? Probably nothing of value. You were titillated. We need to be clear about what we are trying to say to our young people. These programs only create more curiosity and morbid interest.

Secondary prevention programs are those geared toward helping young people already experimenting with drugs to avoid developing drug-related problems resulting from ignorance, arrogance, or immoderate behavior. Kids need our help so they don't:

- get pregnant while high,
- get in cars when the driver has been drinking or drugging,
- ingest dangerous drug combinations,
- freak out on volatile drugs like PCP,
- start dealing drugs.

The key elements of a secondary prevention program are:

1. Sharing of factual drug information
2. Teaching about what drugs do and don't do

3. Exploration of risk factors that lead to drug abuse
4. Frank discussions about peer pressure and conformity
5. Establishing the difference between moderation and abuse
6. Demonstrating ways to handle an emergency situation
7. Exploring alternatives to drugs—nonchemical ways of "turning on" to life and pursuing altered states
8. Creative forums where the kids can talk openly
9. Reaching out to youths in trouble with drugs and other problems
10. Allowing a celebration of youth
11. Developing an ethos of responsibility for one's own body and mind
12. Promoting lifelong practices in good health

The best way to achieve this is for parents and school to work together. In some families these types of issues can be discussed easily; in other families these issues are too hot to handle and need to be addressed in the school setting. That's one reason for making sure the program planning council is comprised of teachers, administrators, students, and parents.

Prevention Program Ideas

Drug Information Library: Available to all students and faculty.

Drug Information Hotline: Gives factual information only. Not a counseling service.

Crisis Intervention Hotline: Gives out drug information and refers callers to available agencies and services.

School Health Fair: Substance misuse is one among other health topics.

Big Brother/Big Sister Program: Kids need healthy role models; older kids befriend and guide younger kids.

Psychodrama and Role Playing: People are growing tired of lectures. Theater using family and adolescent life themes can generate a lot of interest and discussion.

Communication Skills Workshops: Help kids and parents to talk to one another.

Values Clarification Exercises: Stop preaching and help people to creatively formulate and articulate their own values.

Affective Education: Help students to see the powerful role that emotions play in our daily lives.

Sex Education Program: A lot of drug use and misuse occurs around ignorance of our bodies and the relationship between sex and self-image.

Nondrug Ways of Exploring Altered States of Consciousness: This one may take you further than the drug issue. Meditation, running, religious mysticism, yoga—are all fascinating.

Family Life Education Course: Open to parents and students. Can combine didactic (factual) and experiential (exercises) format.

Film Program: Show some good ones and some bad ones and have your audience critique them. Remember, films are only meant to be "triggers" to discussion, not an end in themselves.

Smoking Cessation Program: This is the one that always seems to elude the school setting. You can help kids stop smoking before it becomes a lifelong habit.

Nutrition and Exercise Program: Most kids find "gym" is a drag. Make it more upbeat by helping kids stay trim and eat right through action, not lectures. Junk food may be as harmful as drug abuse.

SOME REALITIES ABOUT DEALING DRUGS

The sale of licit drugs which are controlled substances (can't be obtained without a doctor's prescription—such as Valium) or illicit drugs (illegal by definition—such as heroin) is against the law. That means federal, state, and local ordinances. Laws vary greatly from one part of the country to another, and you need to check this out for your locality. The state police and the local district attorney's office are reliable sources of such information. Even if you think the laws on the books represent "cruel and unusual" punishment or are scientifically inaccurate (how did a hallucinogen like marijuana end up in the same category as heroin or morphine?), your local law-enforcement officials have an obligation to enforce these laws. Some of them do it with relish. In some parts of the country kids and adults end up doing time in jail or prison for a drug offense which would net them only a slap on the wrist in another locale. (See Appendix D for a state-by-state listing of marijuana laws.) Possession of up to seven-eighths of an ounce of marijuana in New York State can only lead to a citation (analogous to a traffic summons) and no criminal record. Try holding that much grass in some southern states and you can end up behind bars and be subject to a stiff fine. However, possess a full ounce or more in New York State and the criminal penalties begin, ranging from misdemeanor to felony depending on the amount and whether or not there was intent to sell. This greater quantity (usually a pound or more of grass, less for other drugs) is called "dealing in weight." Dealing in weight can get you into serious trouble in any state in the Union.

Money or the allure of "free drugs" is the hook that can lead to some big-time headaches for small-time dealers. How do you get free drugs? Consider this from a seventeen-year-old high-school senior:

> It's really easy to keep yourself in free dope, man. Say I buy half a pound of weed [marijuana] for $500. That's eight ounces, right? If I sell seven ounces at $75 per, I take in $525 and I keep one ounce for free and make $25 profit to boot. If I sell the whole eight, I make $100 profit. But I'm not greedy, I just want to keep myself in drugs.

In case someone you know is considering setting up a dealership, consider the sequel:

Things were going along fine for a whole year. I was only selling drugs to people I knew first-hand. I never sold bad stuff. Only quality merchandise—grass and some pills, mostly Quāaludes. You'll never believe what did me in! The cops caught a couple of kids committing vandalism. They were high on beer and ludes. One of the kids, who bought the pills from me, panicked. The cops said if he would tell them where he bought the drugs they would go easy on him. He ratted me out [informed] and the cops nailed me with enough pills in my pocket to get me some heavy time. Some friend!

Drug dealing is big business in America. According to Attorney General William French Smith, gross drug sales nationwide approached $79 billion in 1980, "about equal to the combined profits of America's 500 largest industrial corporations." The illicit marijuana crop in California alone is estimated to be worth in excess of $5 billion. Even lookouts for drug dealers can earn weekly incomes of four to five hundred dollars. The temptations are very real, but it must be kept in mind that the lower down the organizational ladder the drug dealer is, the more vulnerable he is. Middle-class small-time drug dealers don't often appreciate the risks they take when dealing with professional dealers. The *New York Times*[5] told the sad story of Barry S. Weinbaum, a campus drug dealer at Bennington College, whose life was ended at age twenty-two on the Lower East Side of Manhattan; his body was found in a green plastic bag jammed between two decaying buildings. He was dressed in the collegiate clothes that had been his trademark at Bennington. Barry had put himself through school with his earnings from dealing cocaine. The former editor of the college newspaper, captain of the softball team, student of Shakespeare, and proofreader of psychiatric texts met his death traveling in a lethal world of drug dealing in an urban ghetto. Barry wasn't as street-wise as he thought.

Young people rarely understand how frightening it can be to deal with the police. Even when the officers are simply doing their job and not using techniques like entrapment, getting arrested is a real drag. Having their rights read to them, being photographed and fingerprinted, and then having the police call their parents is a shot of reality that anyone can live without.

The police and society in general reserve a special kind of outrage for drug dealers. People are aware that the more drugs are available, the more readily they will be purchased and consumed. Many communities have mounted strong efforts to cut off the supply of drugs coming in. It is certainly true that the really big drug dealers are rarely caught or prosecuted because they hire expensive "dope" lawyers and have some pretty nasty ways of dealing with people who might testify against them. But your local police may be very content to apprehend the small-time dealer. There are several good reasons for this:

1. the law requires them to do so,
2. they are easier to catch and prosecute,
3. the officers may reside in the town where they work and wish to keep drug dealers away from their own families, and
4. arrests lead to promotions.

I have worked with a lot of kids who have been in trouble with the law. Most of them thought the police were "dummies" who busted people only so they could smoke their dope. Experienced officers are very good at this kind of police work and they have some very sophisticated equipment at their disposal. Arresting officers often look like long-distance truck drivers, not cops. These cops are street-wise and love to nail the kid who thinks he can outsmart them.

The trend toward relaxing drug laws so popular during the late 1970s has been halted and may even be reversed. President Carter was seriously considering the decriminalization of marijuana. The Reagan administration shows no similar inclination. With the First Lady's strong interest in the misuse of drugs by the young, it is highly unlikely that any liberalizing trends will be promoted under the present administration in Washington.

Police officers and judges may have a somewhat lenient attitude toward first offenders when the charge involves only simple drug possession. However, they tend to take a much tougher stance when the charge is "possession with the intent to sell" or actual sales. The defendant can forget about saying he was holding it for a friend. No one believes that line anymore. Even if you don't do time or pay a fine (if you are lucky), you will still have a criminal record. If this record includes a felony conviction, it can hurt later on in life. One may find oneself banned from certain professional practices such as law and medicine (the AMA and the ABA have boards of ethics), unable to get bonded, unable to pass security clearances for sensitive positions, and so on. As police records become computerized, it will be easier to keep track of these things, and the likelihood of being haunted forever will increase.

> When I was in college I tried just about every drug known on campus including heroin. As an adult I only do grass and coke. I was the finalist for a very lucrative job with a Fortune 100 firm. They made me take a lie detector test as part of the final phase of interviewing. As soon as the tester asked me "Have you ever used . . . ?" and then went down a long list of drugs, I knew I was doomed. Sure enough, he stopped the test and called in someone from the personnel department who explained that the job was no longer mine.

If you or someone close to you is arrested, remember that you have certain rights under the law. As a general rule, you should say nothing without advice of counsel. Anything you say may be held against you in a court of law. Getting arrested can really shake you up, but you must be indicted and found guilty before the penalty of the law can be brought to bear. If your child is arrested, he or she will need your help. Don't assume guilt until you have heard their side of things—no matter what the arresting officer says. The main object is to get them home and to consult an attorney. Letting them sit in jail overnight to "teach them a lesson" presumes guilt.

The wisest approach is to keep Baretta's warning in mind:

"Don't do the crime if you can't do the time." Stay far away from trafficking in drugs.

HELPING KIDS TO HELP THEMSELVES

The youth drug scene is like a net with large holes. Those kids who experiment with drugs, for the most part, will pass safely through the holes of the net, not experiencing any difficulties with the drugs. Then there are those kids who get caught in the net, turning experimentation into use, into abuse, into addiction. Parents and other adults are usually the last to know. This places young people in a unique position to try to come to the aid of their friends. Now this is a tricky business, and there are no rules. Perhaps by getting away from the notion of everyone "doing their own thing," we as adults can aid our young people, including our own children, to develop a higher sense of social responsibility. Kids try on new fads and friends like clothes. They are doing this at the very same time that they are developing a sense of idealism. Kids have a way of reaching out to one another and caring for their peers. By the time most of us became adults we had successfully learned to turn inward, ignoring the needs of others. The kids today see this and shy away from us as jaded and selfish. But if we come to our children with a sense of caring for their greater community as well as our own, we can place drugs in the context of broader and more enduring issues.

In the following pages you'll find some suggestions for your kids to try out when they want to help their friends. By discussing this advice with your children, you can accomplish a number of important goals:

1. show your kids you realize that drug use occurs in a complicated social context,
2. show them that you care about their friends,
3. model the kind of communication skills you wish to impart to them, and

4. show them you realize that the drug issue is about people, not statistics. (These suggestions, by the way, apply to adult friendships as well.)

Modeling moderation or abstinence: People tend to play follow-the-leader. In many situations kids will be afraid to seem "unhip" and will drink or use drugs even when they don't really want to. This is classic conformity behavior (something we worried about a lot in the 1960s). Help your kids to understand this, and to see that groups need models for abstinence and moderation as well as drunkenness and macho drinking bouts. Doing what you really want requires more maturity and assertiveness than simply aping others' behavior. If just one person says "No" or "Enough for me," this can keep a whole group's drinking or drugging from sinking to the lowest common denominator (usually the person who doesn't know when to stop).

Stating concerns: Parents are often better at this than kids. However, kids do it with fewer games. If someone you know is starting to get into trouble when they drink or drug, what do you do? What would you advise your kids to do? One of the most important questions you can ask someone when trying to diagnose a drug problem is, "Has anyone ever spoken to you about your drug taking?" Often the answer is no. By ignoring people in trouble we enable them to get worse. People who con themselves into believing that they are not in trouble with drugs will only get worse if someone doesn't speak up. It's certainly easy enough to ignore them. If you have any real regard for the person in question, you should state your concern without being judgmental or putting them down. *Say:* "I really worry about you when you have been drinking. Last night everyone was laughing at you and putting you down." *Don't say:* "You are really a fool when you drink. Why don't you wise up and stop drinking!"

What needs to be communicated is responsible concern, the heart of which is this: "I love you but sometimes you do dangerous or silly things. And when you do I will tell you about it because

I care." Help your kids to understand how defensive most adolescents are. ("Don't kick a door down when you can use a key.") On the other hand, if you aren't being heard, you can escalate into a more assertive and hard-hitting statement such as: "I have been trying to reach you and you don't seem to want to hear me. If drinking or drugging is more important to you than honest feedback from a friend, you have a problem. If you want to talk about it I'll be around." This approach requires a lot of patience and can be very frustrating. However, keep these two things in mind:

1. No one is responsible for anyone else's drugging or drinking.
2. You are responsible only for sending the message. The other person is responsible for hearing or not hearing.

Using the "horse" concept. This approach takes stating your concerns a step further. The horse concept goes like this:

If you meet a man on the street and he says, "You are a horse," you scratch your head and wonder if he's nuts. If you continue on and meet a friend who says, "You are a horse," you begin to wonder what is going on. If when you arrive home your sister says, "You are a horse," then you might consider having some hay for dinner.

If the person with the drug problem can't hear you alone, then get some more people who share your perception and concern and speak to him or her in a group. Don't "rat pack" or gang up on your friend with everyone being righteous and talking at the same time. Each person should calmly but firmly state his or her concerns and let your friend know that they wish to help.

Taking a position about your friendship: If your friend is letting drugs come between you, then you have an important choice to make. Kids used to complain to me a lot about what a drag it is to deal with "acid heads" and "Jesus freaks." Their basic complaint is that these kids were capable of relating to people only through drugs or their own brand of Christianity. People want to have a direct relatedness to one another. They don't want any third party getting in the way. If your friends are relating to you only via drugs, then they are not valuing you as a person. You may have to ask them to choose between a meaningful relationship with you and getting high (at least when they are with you). The focus here is on persistent drug use. If the drugs mean that much to them, they aren't ready to have you for a friend. This hurts, but it happens quite often when young people and adults start substituting drugs for people.

Seeking advice: When someone you care about is in trouble with drugs and won't listen to your sound advice, it can be very upsetting to you. Maybe someone else needs to be consulted. Where young people are involved there are two ways to go. One way is to keep your friend's identity hidden. The other is to reveal his or her name. As a parent you would like to feel that your own kids can approach you when they have a concern about themselves or a close friend. You will have to help them to see that sometimes professional help is required. If your own child approaches you about a friend, it is not really necessary for you to know the other child's name. If the drug abuse becomes life-threatening, however, the whole equation may shift radically. How long should anyone wait before volunteering a name? There is no simple answer, but it is clear that most people wait too long. You may have to be willing to put the friendship on the line. To ignore a serious situation which then turns ugly or tragic can lead to a lifetime of guilt. It is commendable that kids will seek advice and then try to use that advice with their friend. But kids have to know that when their best efforts fail, other people must be brought into the picture. If "squealing" saves a life, then it certainly is worthwhile.

Lending an ear: A friend is someone who listens. Sometimes just being a good passive listener can be a release and comfort to a friend. Sometimes we have to be active listeners. Many people use drugs to mask unpleasant or painful feelings or life situations.

102

Try to be there for them when they are not high. If they seem
blue or angry or just plain upset, try to get them to talk it out
with you. If they do it while they are high, try to get them to
talk about it later when they are straight. The task here is to
be not a drug counselor but a hearing and caring friend. A good
tool to use in these situations is called "reflecting feelings." Instead
of making value judgments or giving direct advice, you can say
things like "That must be hard to deal with" or "I'll bet that
makes you feel real sad." These kinds of statements make it
possible for people to open up even more. You can then go on
to share your own feelings and thoughts on the subject.

Drawing the line: One of the toughest things we ever have
to do with people we really care about, like family members or
close friends, is to take a strong position. For example, if you
see someone close to you about to snort some heroin, you will
be right in letting them know what a dumb and dangerous thing
they are about to do and that you want nothing further to do
with them if they must persist in using heroin. And no one who
values their life will travel in a car when the driver is drunk or
stoned—it could end in tragedy. You would be wise to flatly
refuse the ride (and even wiser not to permit that person to
drive at all). Or if you find out that your friend is spending all
his or her money on cocaine and wants to borrow some from
you, you would be wise to turn them down.

Turning on to life (without drugs): Happiness is a lull between
disasters. Even the most powerful feelings of ecstasy are usually
quite short-lived. We keep trying to make "sense out of nonsense."
All of us are born with a wonderful capacity to experience life
emotionally. Sense is the use of the central nervous system for
rational thought. Why do we prohibit using that same mechanism
for feeling our emotions (nonsense)? People keep using drugs
to get to various states of feeling because we are uptight about
expressing and sharing our emotions. Almost all the drug addicts
and alcoholics I have known have problems in the area of feelings.
Only when they are able to learn to handle these feelings is a

drug-free life possible. This means that prevention efforts must address themselves to the social and emotional life of young people if they are to work. Teaching young people to express and talk out their feelings is the ounce of prevention we should be pursuing, instead of lectures on pharmacology. Want to get high without drugs? Try some of the following:

- run across an open field or along a beach
- ask one of your grandparents what life is about
- play with a baby
- give a friend a gift that you made with your own hands
- work hard at something and see it through to completion
- learn to meditate
- stop eating junk food
- write some poetry for yourself (it doesn't have to rhyme)
- climb a mountain
- say thank you more often
- beat the shit out of a pillow the next time you are really angry
- stop biting your nails (or shed another bad habit)
- read a good book (later for the comic books or video games)
- give someone a real long hug
- call your father at work and tell him you love him
- have a good cry about that thing you have been hiding for too long

Feels good just thinking about some of these things, right? The next time you want to get high just ask yourself if the drugs are really necessary. But drugs or not, don't expect to hold on to the feeling for very long. That's how emotions are. They run like a river—from streams to oceans. Don't push the river, flow with it!

Our society is the play-it-safe crowd. We don't seem to want to get involved anymore. We don't want to be hurt. But this is unrealistic—having your feelings hurt is part of living. Like stress, it is unavoidable. If you want to have friends and be intimate with people, you have to take chances. This is the message we must give our young people if we are going to teach them to help others. Showing responsible concern to friends is not easy, but it makes for enduring and more meaningful relationships. The best way to teach your kids is to be a good model yourself. By following the suggestions made in this chapter in the context of school life and combining them with material from the chapter on the family, you will have a good, constructive link between the two places where children spend most of their time.

CHAPTER THREE

Drugs and the Workplace

I was using speed to wake me up and keep me going during the workday. I used downs [barbiturates] and alcohol to get me to sleep at night. The diet pills I took had some more speed in them. I liked to smoke grass and do some cocaine on the weekends. Once in a while I would drop a lude to mellow me out. It got to be a real hassle at work. I have a responsible job and the drugs were getting in the way. It's a full-time job just balancing all the drugs. Sometimes I would forget things and really get disorganized. Eventually I could not keep it all together. So I took a holiday from drugs and everything has been a lot calmer.

—VICE PRESIDENT, *Fortune 500 company*

The kids who came up through the counterculture of the 1960s and early '70s have entered the work force. Whether introduced to drugs during the days of campus protest or in the rice paddies of Vietnam, a whole generation of young people have grown into their maturity for whom drugs were very much a part of that maturing process. Drugs that used to be found among students, musicians, street people, and other fringe groups within society have made their way into the workplace. Mainstream America is turning on. The sweet smell of marijuana is now emanating from corporate boardrooms, typing pools, assembly lines, and union meeting halls. Drugs have become a fact of life in working America. There are many reasons why people use drugs at work:

- to counteract boredom
- to counteract fatigue
- to energize themselves
- to deal with pressure and tension
- to tune out on work
- to get through the workday
- to tranquilize and calm themselves
- to facilitate business deals
- to make extra money selling drugs at work
- to put themselves in a creative frame of mind
- to show off (especially status drugs like cocaine)
- to counteract "burnout"
- to self-medicate against depression and anxiety
- to be more outgoing
- to stay awake
- to shut off nonwork stimuli
- to forget about troubles

This is only a partial list. There are almost as many reasons as there are people using drugs. Some people take drugs as a planned act. Others take drugs without conceiving of their actions as "drug taking"; examples of this are smoking cigarettes, drinking coffee, and the use of alcohol. Some people actively seek to get high while at work. Others take medications, both prescription and OTC (over the counter), to deal with any number of physical symptoms and maladies. (Over $500 million a year is spent on cold remedies alone, and $5 billion a year in wages and productivity are lost due to the common cold.) Few people realize that food acts as a mood changer and happily eat their way through millions of business breakfasts, lunches, and dinners each year, altering their emotional states at work.

There are powerful emotional biases at work when people discuss drugs. Very few people have a neutral attitude. They tend to be defensive, judgmental, argumentative, condescending, proselytizing, grandiose, all-knowing, righteous. People who use drugs all have their own drug(s) of choice and tend to look askance at the next person's choices. In the words of one college student:

> My grandfather had his home-grown wine, my father likes his Scotch, my mother digs martinis and I like grass and hash. It's all the same shit. Man, we are all just trying to get high. It seems when I try to talk about this with my folks that one person's drug is another person's poison. I wish everyone would be a little more honest about what's really going down.

And in the words of a middle-management insurance executive:

> The big bosses down a lot of booze during lunch and after hours. The girls in the secretarial pool like to smoke pot. My colleagues and I enjoy a little coke after work and sometimes we do it when we have to work long hours and meet a deadline. God only knows what drugs the file clerks are doing.

None of these people are addicted. They manage to use drugs in a manner they feel is safe and fun and even productive (at work). They are quick to defend their drugs of choice and can rhapsodize about them for hours. Alcohol has not had to give way to the newer drugs, which have simply been added to the list. Whether your preference is for a brandy alexander or a line of coke, you are chemically altering your consciousness.

The United States Armed Forces constitutes a significant proportion of the American work force, with some 3 million active-duty soldiers and another 3 million military dependents. The military estimates that the equivalent of four battalions of infantry a year are unavailable for duty because of drug-related problems (the soldiers are in jail or in treatment). A Department of Defense worldwide survey[1] of active-duty personnel reported that about 83 percent drank occasionally and 21 percent indicated a heavy beer-drinking pattern (eight or more drinks in a single day at least monthly during the past twelve months). The same survey reported that although the highest prevalence of drinking any alcohol was recorded by senior officers, heavy drinking was reported almost exclusively by enlisted personnel. It is estimated that the cost of lost production to the military due to alcohol abuse is $410 million annually. When a jet plane crashed on the deck of the *USS Nimitz* it was discovered that six out of ten crew members had evidence of recent marijuana use in their bodies. While teaching a course on alcoholism counseling to a group of noncommissioned officers at West Point, I was told:

> Whether you drink or drug has a lot to do with where you are stationed. A tour in Korea is viewed as a drinking man's tour, as the Korean government takes a hard line against drug use. A tour in Europe, especially West Germany, means easy access to a wide variety of drugs including hashish and heroin. I've been all over the world in this man's army and I've seen just about every form of drug use and abuse imaginable.

Vietnam-era veterans strongly resent the stereotype that they are all either drug addicts or alcoholics or walking time bombs ready to commit violent acts against civilians. These men know that a lot of heavy-duty drinking and drugging went on in Vietnam and that some of them came home with a drug problem that required active treatment. But they also know that most of the troops who drank and drugged in Vietnam did not bring the problem home. Studies have shown a surprisingly high remission rate even for heroin addiction, without benefit of treatment. This is true despite the fact that some vets suffer from post-traumatic delayed-stress syndrome and use drugs and alcohol as a self-administered form of relief. One soldier put it this way:

When you are in an insane place like 'Nam you do insane things just to get from day to day. Getting stoned was just another way of counting off the days and passing time between missions until you finished your tour and went back to the world [home].

A practical problem faced by many veterans has been that prospective employers fear they may be undependable because they served in a war that has left them psychological casualties. If there is one thing that a person recovering from addiction needs to ensure that recovery, it is a job. It is essential for a sense of personal and family dignity, as well as for paying the bills.

There are some 13 million alcoholics and problem drinkers in America. Only about 5 percent of these men and women can be found on skid row. The other 12,350,000 are people just like you and me. A $450 million private (profit-making) alcoholism treatment network has grown up to serve the 10 percent of corporate America who can't handle their alcohol. It is also estimated that two-thirds of the drug and alcohol abuse in business and industry is suppressed. Traditionally the drug alcohol has had the greatest degree of acceptance in American society, and therefore in the commerce and industry of that society. It was once common for workers to have a drink on the job (the "4 o'clock dram"). To the extent that the captains of industry tend to predate the newer drugs, they tend to frown upon them. To the extent that your boss is young enough or "hip" enough to have been exposed to coke, grass, and hashish, he or she will probably use them in secret (public espousal would spell condemnation). But the other drugs are coming up from the underground in offices and factories all over America. Workers at all levels, including supervisors, are developing an "emotional radar system" with which they seek out kindred souls in drug use. Most of the cues are subtle, but a certain word used here or there or a phrase unique to the drug culture is a real clue to who is using and who isn't. Don't be fooled by traditional stereotypes. Drug use, just like alcohol use, is becoming very democratic. You don't need long hair or dark glasses or to speak in street slang to appreciate the effects of many drugs. The fellow in the vested suit and rep tie is just as likely to be getting high as the more obvious counterculture types.

As much as 10 percent of the national work force is suffering from alcoholism or problem drinking. The most current official estimates are that alcoholism and problem drinking are causing a loss to American society of $50–60 billion a year. Alcohol abuse and alcoholism feature prominently in lost productivity and sales, health and medical costs, industrial accidents, absenteeism, lateness, grievances, training, and termination costs. Alcoholism also figures prominently in rape, assault, murder, child molesting, child abuse and neglect, spouse abuse and other domestic violence, suicide, automobile accidents, and automobile accident deaths.

More on the Impact of Alcoholism in Industry

1. Nationally, an average of 6 percent of all employees suffer from alcoholism and 4 percent from problem drinking, causing a majority of labor-management problems such as:
   - The alcoholic employee is absent two to four times more often than the nonalcoholic employee.
   - On-the-job accidents to alcoholic employees are two to four times more frequent than among nonalcoholic employees. Off-the-job accidents are four to six times more frequent.
   - Sickness and accident benefits paid out for alcoholic employees are three times greater than for the average nonalcoholic employee.
   - In one assembly plant, out of 746 grievances filed during one year, 48.6 percent were alcohol related.
2. It is conservatively estimated that each alcoholic employee costs a company the equivalent of 25 percent of his or her salary.
3. The annual cost to American industry is in excess of $11 billion.
4. An undetermined percentage of employees are seriously affected by an alcoholism problem in their family.

Drugs in the workplace cost businesses in increased absenteeism, poor work performance, thefts, accidents, wasted time, and higher insurance rates. Negative consequences to the employee include industrial accidents, failure to be promoted, lost time and pay, bad references, loss of job, and a criminal record (if arrested on the job for illicit drug possession or sale). The American work force is involved in significant rates of regular drug use in all occupational groups except farming.

Heroin addicts can and do hold down paying jobs, are hard to detect, and commit a wide variety of crimes at the work site. Here are some of the "scams" that addicts run in the work setting:[2]

auto mechanic	steals parts and tools
clothing machine operator	steals coats by placing them in the garbage and picking them up after hours
phone installer	falsifies installation orders and sells phones to customers at one-half price
stock clerk	steals negotiable bonds, forges an I.D. and cashes bonds at local bank
medical assistant	steals drugs and syringes
credit collector	steals cash payments
air conditioning installer	steals tools and parts, burgles customers' apartments
steel-mill worker	wholesales large quantities of marijuana in an abandoned section of the plant
pharmacy clerk	steals prescriptions

dry-cleaning-store worker	gives customer receipts to friends who claim the customers' clothing
secretary	steals money from co-workers' purses
supermarket worker	steals meat ("cattle rustling") and sells it in the neighborhood at half-price
truck driver	steals from workers' lockers
nurse's aide	steals syringes and other medical supplies
messenger	steals cash from employer

I have worked with a number of corporate officers who used far more elaborate and sophisticated schemes to steal money from their companies, all to feed a drug habit (heroin or cocaine). I treated a young man who sold both stocks and drugs on the floor of the New York Stock Exchange. I also treated a college registrar who used a computer terminal to secure student loans for fictitious students, all to support his cocaine use. Working addicts are more similar to other workers than they are to nonworking addicts. For example, they tend to be older, better educated, more often married, and are more likely to be white than nonworking addicts. Despite their heroin habits, more than half hold their jobs for a year or more.

RISE AND SHINE

Can you guess what drug these people are talking about?

I can't get started without it. I'm no good to anyone until I have some!

Every time I need a lift I take some; it really energizes me.

Some times when I've had too much I really feel wired and a little crazy. Like I can't sit still, or stop talking, and I'm constantly running to the bathroom.

The more I have in the morning, the less I feel like having lunch.

I would never have gotten through my final exams in college without it.

Have you guessed yet? Symptoms of usage in many people are virtually indistinguishable from an anxiety condition. Here is some more information that may help.[3]

MYSTERY-DRUG SYMPTOMS:

irritability

nervousness

nausea

vomiting

diarrhea

epigastric pain (*in region over the pit of the stomach*)

diuresis (*abnormal secretion of urine*)

flushing

arrhythmias (*irregular heartbeat*)

sensory disturbance

insomnia

tremulousness

agitation

palpitations

headaches

ringing in the ears

visual flashes of light

delayed sleep onset

frequent sleep interruption

SIGNS THAT DOCTORS LOOK FOR:

tachypnea (*abnormal rapidity of breathing*)

reflex hyperexcitability

muscle twitching

hyperesthesia (*increased sensitivity to touch*)

extrasystoles (*premature contractions of one of the parts of the heart*)

tachycardia (*abnormal rapidity of the heart*)

arrhythmias (*irregular heartbeat*)

WITHDRAWAL SIGNS INCLUDE:

headache

nervousness

irritability

lethargy

restlessness

drowsiness and excessive yawning

dysphoria (*opposite of euphoria*)

disinclination to work

inability to concentrate

nausea

runny nose

Answer: The drug is *caffeine!* You have just read a description of the symptoms and signs of caffeinism, or "coffee-drinker's syndrome," the name given to chronic caffeine intoxification. People who suffer from caffeinism have a history of drinking a lot of coffee (five to ten cups a day) or other products containing caffeine.

Sixty percent of American adults drink an average of more than two cups of coffee per day; 25 percent drink five or more cups a day; and 10 percent drink seven or more cups a day. It takes about 50 to 100 milligrams of caffeine to produce the characteristic pharmacologic action of the drug. Many people consume enough caffeine each day to produce symptoms of caffeinism with-

Caffeine Found in Foods and Drugs

Source	Caffeine (milligrams)
BEVERAGES	
Coffee (5 ounces)	
Drip method	146
Percolated	110
Instant regular	53
Decaffeinated	2
Tea (5 ounces) (loose or in tea bags)	
1-minute brew	9–33
3-minute brew	20–46
5-minute brew	20–50
Iced tea, can (12 ounces)	22–36
Cocoa and Chocolate	
Cocoa (made from mix), 6 ounces	10
Milk chocolate, 1 ounce	6
Baking chocolate, 1 ounce	35
*Soda (12-ounce cans)**	
Diet Mr. Pibb	52
Mountain Dew	52
Mello Yellow	51
Tab	44
Shasta Cola	42
Dr Pepper	38
Diet Dr Pepper	37
Pepsi Cola	37
Royal Crown Cola	36
Diet Rite Cola	34
Diet Pepsi	34
Coca-Cola	34
Mr. Pibb	33
Cragmore Cola	Trace
7-Up	0
Sprite	0
Diet 7-Up	0
RC-100	0

Source	Caffeine (milligrams)
BEVERAGES	
Diet Sunkist Orange	0
Sunkist Orange	0
Patio Orange	0
Fanta Orange	0
Fresca	0
Hires Root Beer	0
NONPRESCRIPTION DRUGS (STANDARD DOSE)	
Stimulants	
Caffedrine capsules	200
NoDoz tablets	200
Vivarin tablets	200
Pain Relievers	
Anacin	64
Excedrin	130
Midol	65
Plain aspirin	0
Tylenol	0
Diuretics	
Aqua-Ban	200
Permathene H_2Off	200
Pre-Mens Forte	100
Cold Remedies	
Coryban-D	30
Dristan	32
Triaminicin	30
Weight-control aids	
Dexatrim	200
Dietac	200
Promaline	280

* As tested by Consumers Union for October 1981 issue of *Consumer Reports;* formulations may change.

Source: *Consumer Reports,* October 1981, © Consumers Union of the United States, Inc.

117

out consciously realizing it. A child who consumes a lot of chocolate (there are about 25 milligrams per small bar) and cola soft drinks (or others containing caffeine—see the table) runs the same risks of caffeinism due to his lower body weight.

Caffeine belongs to a class of drugs called methylxanthines. The three main drugs found in this class are caffeine, theobromine (found in chocolate milk and cocoa), and theophylline. Decaffeinated coffee contains a small amount of caffeine (about 2 milligrams) and some theobromine and theophylline.

Among heavy users, the drug caffeine causes physical dependence, with withdrawal symptoms and craving. Heroin addicts in both drug-free and methadone-maintenance treatment programs drink an inordinate amount of coffee, up to twenty cups per day. And they will add 3 to 5 teaspoons of sugar to each cup of coffee. This looks like symptom substitution to many in the field who are concerned about switched addictions. These addicts were barely detoxified from heroin before they had already adopted a new drug habit. When I directed the Alcoholism Treatment Program at Beth Israel Medical Center in New York City, we served only decaffeinated coffee to our patients. This was done to eliminate the mood-altering effects of coffee and to prevent gastritis and stomach ulcers so often found in alcoholics.

Caffeine has no nutritional value and only about 5 calories per cup. However, when you add a teaspoon of sugar (15 to 25 calories) and a teaspoon of cream (another 30 calories), you can see how coffee drinking can add to your waistline.

There is a growing controversy about the relative safety of caffeine. There exist a number of presumptive links, based on several studies, between caffeine and a number of serious health problems. Everyone agrees that caffeine stimulates the central nervous system, can constrict blood vessels and speed up the heart, and stimulates the brain, stomach, kidneys, ovaries, and testes. For many people caffeine's action is similar to another stimulant drug—methamphetamine, known as "speed." It first lifts you up and then sets you down, sometimes with depressed feelings. As caffeine causes a rise and fall of blood sugar levels it can lead to symptoms commonly found in hypoglycemia (low blood sugar) such as fatigue, lethargy, and depression.

Joan's Story

Joan had been in and out of psychotherapy over a period of seven years. Diagnosed as suffering from an "anxiety neurosis" by other therapists, she could not understand why all the money she had spent on therapy had not brought her some significant relief. Her family doctor gave her a clean bill of health and suggested she was suffering from "nerves," which led to her first therapy referral. Although the doctor asked her about drinking and drugs it never occurred to him to ask her about her coffee drinking. Fortunately for Joan, she gave herself away in our first session together. She had brought a thermos full of steaming hot coffee! She complained to me of chronic nervousness, periodic bouts of depression, and years of sleep disturbance. All this despite her happy marriage, a rewarding job, and two lovely children. Her doctor had, of course, prescribed a tranquilizer for her "nerves." On workdays Joan drank about twelve to fifteen cups of coffee, and twenty per day on weekends. She had no idea that she had a serious drug problem. I asked her why she brought the thermos of coffee, and she answered that she was nervous and that the coffee helped to relax her. When I explained to her about caffein addiction, it took only two sessions for her to understand and accept what had been happening to her. She did taper off slowly and then switched to decaffeinated coffee. About a month later she had a "slip" and began sneaking more regular coffee. A referral to Pills Anonymous (P.A.) gave Joan the added group support she needed to deal with her drug craving. Today she drinks only drug-free herbal tea and feels much better. This time the total cost of therapy was $250 (P.A. is free). The previous missed diagnosis had cost Joan thousands of dollars in unnecessary therapy.

According to Dr. Sanford Miller, director of the Food and Drug Administration's Bureau of Foods, caffeine is "a potent biologically active material." The FDA is seriously considering two actions at this time: one is the removal of caffeine from its list of "Generally Recognized as Safe (GRAS)" list of food additives, and the second is to eliminate the present requirement that cola drinks contain caffeine. The FDA is taking the position that more needs to be known. Dr. Miller states the agency's position on caffeine (April 1982): "We are not saying it's unsafe, we're just not saying it's safe." Our current concern over caffeine began in 1978 when an advisory committee to the FDA reported that too much caffeine might have a deleterious effect on central-nervous-system development. Since then several studies have linked the drug with birth defects, fibrocystic breast disease (a nonmalignant disorder), and pancreatic cancer.

Researchers from the Boston Collaborative Drug Surveillance Program surveyed hospital patients who had had a coronary and those who had been admitted for other conditions. They found that men and women who drank more than four cups of coffee a day were twice as likely to have a heart attack as those who abstained from it. The fly in the ointment may be the variable of cigarette smoking. According to Dr. Jean Mayer, president of Tufts University and one of America's leading nutrition experts: "While there is a correlation between coffee drinking and cigarette smoking, the reasons for the relationship between coffee drinking and heart attacks remain a mystery." Other studies have suggested an association between coffee drinking and bladder cancer. Again, the villain here may be the association between coffee drinking and cigarette smoking, as a causal relationship between smoking and bladder cancer has been established.

Children who consume six cans of cola per day or the equivalent (in chocolate candy, for instance) become jumpy and speak faster than normal. Adults who consume the same amount of caffeine (about 300 milligrams) have more subjective reactions, such as mood changes.

Because of the possibility of birth defects, more and more doctors are advising abstinence and certainly moderation (no more than two cups or equivalent per day) for pregnant women. In September 1980 Dr. Jere Goyan, then FDA commissioner, said that a pregnant woman should "put caffeine on her list of unnecessary substances which she should avoid." Scientists at Harvard

University studied the effects of coffee drinking in more than 12,000 women and reported their results in the January 1982 issue of the *New England Journal of Medicine.* They found no detectable ill effects on the unborn babies caused by caffeine, but they did find defects caused by cigarette smoking.

In 1981 an editorial appeared in the medical journal *Lancet,* which said that *moderate* coffee drinking had not been definitively shown to cause any harm and recommended that those who enjoyed it should probably continue. According to the *Book of Health,* published by the American Health Foundation, "Used in *moderation* [emphasis added], it [coffee] is not harmful to most people." Dr. Mayer states:

> In the meantime, what is the coffee drinker to do? The answer, I think, is *moderation* [emphasis added]. Coffee drinking can become excessive—up to ten or fifteen cups a day. And if all that coffee contains cream and sugar, the caloric intake can be substantial. It is not unreasonable to set five cups as an upper limit.

Doses are usually described for the "average" person. "Average" or "normal" is a statistical concept and many of us deviate from the norm. Don't worry about your friends who can consume lots of coffee or cola without negative effects. If you are experiencing negative effects from caffeine, all it means is that your body can't handle that drug. Your body is trying to tell you something important and you should be listening.

The next time the coffee wagon comes around in your office, stop and ask yourself, How is this drug affecting me? Do I want the effect? Do I need the effect? Should I modify my intake of caffeine? One way to find out if you are addicted to caffeine is to stop using it for two full days. If you experience any of the withdrawal symptoms listed earlier, then you will know that you are hooked. If you can continue cold turkey, fine, but some of you may find you need to taper off more slowly. The withdrawal symptoms usually come on eighteen hours after your last dose of the drug. They can last from a few days to several weeks.

All that is required to make the symptoms disappear is another dose of caffeine. But then you'd be hooked again.

The choice is yours. There are four alternatives available to you when it comes to caffeine: abstinence, moderation, heavy use, or addiction.

How to Reduce Your Caffeine Habit

1. First try the two-day no-caffeine test to see if you need to cut back. Or you may decide without going through withdrawal that it's time to cut back or quit.

2. Do *not* use tranquilizers to deal with the jitters of withdrawal, or you may end up with another kind of drug problem. They'll pass when the withdrawal is completed. Stay away from sleeping pills as well.

3. Avoid medications, either prescription or OTC, that contain caffeine. (The label on OTC drugs will tell you if caffeine is an ingredient.) If you want to cut out all stimulants, be sure to avoid all the methylxanthines (theobromine and theophylline). Some prescription drugs that contain caffeine are Cafergot, Migralam, Migral tablets, Fiorinal, Eggic, Apectol, Soma Compound and Darvon Compound.

4. Stay away from sodas that contain caffeine (see the table for a list of some that don't).

5. Start cutting back on the amount of coffee you drink. You may want to switch to decaffeinated coffee right away. You can also mix Decaf with regular coffee, gradually reducing the proportions until it's all Decaf. Coffees blended with grain or chicory have less caffeine.

6. Avoid that second cup of coffee. If you are thirsty, drink something else.

7. Switch to drug-free herbal teas. If diet isn't a big concern, switch to low-fat milk, fruit juices, or just plain water. One of my patients does very nicely with club soda with a twist of lemon.

8. Coffee drinkers find they miss that early-morning lift. Do your body and your mind a big favor: get into some good cardiovas-

---

cular exercise instead—jogging, aerobics, calisthenics. Some people use meditation to achieve a state of "relaxed energy" first thing in the a.m.

9. You will experience some craving. This is due to both physical and psychological dependency. Talk it out with someone and don't give in to it. If no one is around, call someone and have them keep you straight until the desire wanes.

AMERICA'S NICOTINE BLUES

Ivan's story

He had been smoking cigarettes since his late teens. At age thirty-four he discovered that he had coronary artery disease. It had advanced so far that triple-bypass surgery was necessary to save his life. The operation was a success, and his mother, his wife, his two sons, and other relatives and friends were relieved. Despite warnings from his surgeon and his cardiologist, he returned to cigarette smoking as soon as the postoperative pain had passed. He has all the insight in the world about his smoking problem. He says he can't shake the addiction. His wife isn't much help, as she smokes too. He knows that smoking is one of the major risk factors in the development of coronary artery disease. His prognosis could turn out to be grim.

Cigarette smokers have something in common with heroin addicts, speed freaks, garbage heads, and alcoholics: their addiction is a way of life. Smokers overdose (burning in the chest, extreme dizziness, vomiting, loss of appetite), they go through some heavy-duty withdrawal (extreme irritability, intense craving, sleepless-ness, distractibility, obsessive talking about smoking), and generally tend to adopt behaviors that go along with any addiction: protecting their supply, borrowing money or cigarettes, sneaking cigarettes, lying to themselves and others about stopping, feeling they can't enjoy life without their drug, and using all the other rationalizations and defenses needed to explain away a dangerous and life-threatening habit. Smokers learn to ignore the pleas of loved ones, they learn to deny their own objective medical symptoms, blaming them on other causes, they learn to lie and manipulate, they often invade other people's (nonsmokers') space and rights, they avoid medical checkups for fear of hearing bad news (often missing an opportunity to deal with various illnesses in their earliest stages), and so on.

Tobacco use has been around for centuries. First discovered by explorers among the natives in the Americas, it was brought to England around 1592 by Sir Walter Raleigh. Sailors and traders planted tobacco seeds along their trade routes to ensure ample supplies (you see, they knew about craving even back then).

In the United States, the annual per capita consumption of cigarettes was just under 100 in 1910, up to 400 by 1920, and up to 1,000 by 1930. During World War II, cigarette smoking became extremely popular, particularly among men. This was due in part to the mass manufacturing of cigarettes, which brought the price down. By the 1970s, men and women together smoked a per capita average of 4,100 cigarettes a year. Many male smokers have stopped, while many women have just started. Today the proportion of adult smokers is about the same in both sexes—about 36 percent of both men and women. That's about 60 million smokers! In dollars, retail expenditures for cigarettes increased from an estimated $7.2 billion in 1964 (the year the surgeon general's first warnings on the dangers of smoking came out) to an estimated $10.5 billion in 1970—an increase of 45 percent.

We commonly think of nicotine—the primary hazardous and addicting ingredient in cigarettes, cigars, pipe tobacco, and snuff—as a stimulant. However, it can act as a depressant or tranquilizer as well. Pharmacologically speaking, nicotine is a liquid alkaloid, freely soluble in water. It turns brown on exposure to air and is the chief alkaloid found in tobacco. It has no therapeutic use and has been discarded by modern medicine. Nicotine can stimulate the central nervous system, especially the medullary centers (respiratory, emetic, and vasomotor). This stimulation is followed by depression, and repeated administration of nicotine causes tolerance (you need more of the drug to get the original effect).

The litany of physical damage wrought by smoking is awesome. Here are some of the facts, according to the American Cancer Society.

Fact: Smokers subject themselves to a much greater risk of death or disability at a young age. The death rate of cigarette smokers at all ages is higher than that of nonsmokers. It climbs in proportion to the number of cigarettes smoked, the number of years the person has smoked, and the earlier the age at which they started. Smoking will cause about 130,000 deaths from cancer this year. It is the major cause of cancers of the lung, larynx, oral cavity, and esophagus, and a contributory factor to cancers of the bladder, kidneys, and pancreas. Quitting smoking reduces the risk of cancer.

Fact: Men who smoke less than half a pack a day have a death rate about 60 percent higher than that of nonsmokers; a pack to two packs a day, about 90 percent higher; and two or more packs a day, 120 percent higher.

Fact: Cigarette smoking is one of the major risk factors in heart attacks (others include high blood pressure, obesity, and high blood cholesterol). Cigarette smokers have 70 percent more heart attacks than nonsmokers. When other risk factors are also present, the risk goes up greatly. Cigarette smokers have an abnormally high number of strokes.

Fact: Lung cancer is rare among nonsmokers but is the most frequent cause of death among cigarette smokers after heart attacks and strokes, and is directly related to the number of cigarettes smoked. It is estimated that 85 percent of lung cancers are caused by smoking, causing some 100,000 deaths per year in the United States.

Fact: Deaths from emphysema and chronic bronchitis—lingering diseases which cause suffering for years—increased by 550 percent in the thirty years from 1945 to 1975. Most of those who died were smokers. The more cigarettes smoked, the greater the likelihood of disease. The smoker's risk of death from emphysema and chronic bronchitis is from 6½ to 15 times that of the nonsmoker.

Fact: Male cigarette smokers have about five times the normal risk of dying of mouth cancer. Larynx cancer is six to nine times as frequent among cigarette smokers as among nonsmokers; a smoker's chance of dying from this cancer is four to five times that of a nonsmoker. Deaths from urinary bladder cancer are two to three times as numerous among cigarette smokers as among nonsmokers. Smokers are also more likely to get pancreatic cancer.

Fact: The lung cancer rate of women has doubled in ten years and will eventually equal that of men. Pregnant women who smoke have a greater number of stillbirths than nonsmoking women; and their infants are more likely to die within the first month. Their babies more often weigh less than 5½ pounds— which is considered premature—and are exposed to more risk of disease and death. Women who abstain from smoking while pregnant protect their own health and that of their baby.

Fact: Cigarettes are the cause of more than one-third of all residential fire deaths, according to the United States Fire Administration. In 1981 smoking materials ignited 63,518 homes, caused $305 million in property damage, injured 3,819 people and killed 2,144 others. Congress and a growing number of state legislatures are considering requiring cigarettes that would not burn long enough or hot enough to ignite materials like bedding or upholstery. Cigarette manufacturers are opposing such legislation.

Fact: Sidestream smoke—the smoke inhaled by nonsmokers who are near smokers—is a possible serious health problem.

Fact: Ninety-five percent of those who have quit have done it without organized programs. Stopping "cold turkey" appears to be more effective than cutting down gradually.

Fact: "Brief and simple" advice from a doctor is potentially the most cost-effective way of getting smokers to quit. Smoking prevention programs for young people should stress the social and immediate effects of smoking rather than the long-term medical consequences.

After reading a list like this you can see that addictive behavior is almost completely irrational. Surgeon General C. Everett Koop stated that "cigarette smoking is clearly identified as the chief preventable cause of death in our society," and he declared in 1982 that smoking is "the most important health issue of our time." Denial, rationalization, intellectualization, and other ego defense mechanisms allow smokers to continue smoking with the conviction that these terrible things can "never happen to me."

Are You a Nicotine Junkie?

- Your breath stinks! Do people rarely want to kiss your mouth or stand close to you during conversations?
- Your clothes, hair, fingers, and the drapes and other things in your home or office probably smell pretty awful as well. You can't tell because you became inured to the smell a long time ago.
- You are being perceived by a lot of other people, including your boss, as a compulsive junkie!
- What about your wind? When you play ball or golf or bowl do you find yourself gasping for breath?
- How many people avoid you and your office because they can't stand the smoke? More than you think!
- It's embarrassing when you run out of cigarettes. An otherwise healthy and well-adjusted adult is transformed into a very uptight and nervous person when you have a "nicotine fit."

- What color are your teeth? A close look in the mirror may reveal some strange colors.
- How many times have you burned holes in your clothes or an important document? Ever started a fire in your boss's or a client's ashtray?
- Are your clothes full of ashes? your desk? your bed?
- Do you find that you are running to the bathroom a lot? Nicotine can cause excessive urination and diarrhea.
- Did it ever occur to you that the macho (or macha) image you are trying to project with that cigarette really isn't impressing anyone? It's your own fantasy.

One of the highlights of the 1982 *Surgeon General's Report on Smoking* is the concern regarding sidestream smoke. This is the smoke emitted from smoldering tobacco in a steady stream. Smoke particles and ingredients are found in higher concentrations in sidestream than in mainstream smoke, the smoke drawn directly from the mouthpiece of a tobacco product during active puffing. The authors and sponsors of the 1982 report have urged nonsmokers to avoid inhaling cigarette smoke, even though the link between such passive or involuntary smoking and cancer is still a matter of scientific debate. Two studies, in Greece and Japan, have found an elevated and statistically significant incidence of lung cancer among the nonsmoking wives of smoking husbands. Avoid secondhand smoke whenever possible.

There appear to be special dangers for those who combine cigarette smoking with the consumption of alcohol. A great deal of statistical evidence has been gathered which shows that the risks of cigarette smoking are increased when the smoker also drinks alcoholic beverages. One study analyzed the chemicals in the breath of people while they smoked, while they drank, and while they did both at about the same time. When the subjects both sipped and puffed, a chemical called ethyl nitrite appeared in detectable amounts in the breath. It did not matter whether the drink preceded the smoking or vice versa, as long as they were reasonably close together. Ethyl nitrite is known to produce mutations in living cells. Such mutagens are often also carcino-genic (cancer causing). Neither smoking alone nor drinking alone produced detectable amounts of the chemical in the breath. Booze and smoke appear to be a deadly combination.

In recent years smokers have sought to derive health benefits by switching to reduced-tar brands of cigarettes. According to the National Academy of Sciences, smokers who switch to low-tar, low-nicotine cigarettes are not decreasing their chances of lung cancer because they tend to puff and inhale more. Therefore the possible health benefits are doubtful. Smokers of low-tar brands may unconsciously inhale more deeply and hold the smoke in their lungs longer to satisfy their craving for nicotine. The problem is that "most heavy smokers, regardless of brand, tend to maintain high nicotine levels." Interestingly these findings of the National Academy of Sciences contradict a similar study recently released by the American Cancer Society. The ACS study showed a 26 percent lower mortality rate from lung cancer in smokers of low-tar, low-nicotine cigarettes when compared with those who smoked high-tar, high-nicotine brands.

Of course the Tobacco Institute, which represents manufactur-ers of tobacco products, continues to contend that the question is "still open" on whether smoking causes cancer. The surgeon general dismissed that contention, saying, "The evidence is strong and scientific and we stand by it."

One of the common excuses for continuing to smoke is the notion that smoking will relax you and get you through times that are stressful. This can become a deadly rationalization be-cause stress, in its scientific sense, is an unavoidable part of life. This would then sentence the smoker to a lifetime of carcinogenic behavior. Let's take a closer look at the real nature of this often used but poorly understood concept of human stress. According to Dr. Hans Selye, a leading world expert on the subject:[4]

- Stress is the nonspecific response of the body to any de-mand made upon it.

- It doesn't matter whether the agent or situation we face is pleasant or unpleasant; what counts is the intensity of the demand for readjustment or adaptation.
- Stress is more than nervous tension.
- Stress is not always the cause of damage. Any amount of normal activity—a game of chess or a passionate embrace—can produce considerable stress without causing harmful effects. Damaging or unpleasant stress is "distress."
- Stress is not always something to be avoided. In fact, it cannot be completely avoided.
- Complete freedom from stress is death.

To be alive is to face stress—each and every day of our lives. How we respond to it and whether or not we are flexible in the face of it is what really matters. According to Dr. Selye we react to all stress through a biological mechanism which he calls the "general adaptation syndrome." It consists of three stages: an alarm reaction (the stimulus grabs our attention), the stage of resistance (in which we actively contend with the stimulus through either "fight" or "flight"), and a stage of exhaustion (during which we rest and replenish ourselves). You are kidding yourself if you think you can ever reach a point where you won't be under stress and therefore not "need" a cigarette to "calm you down." By using smoking to contend with stress you are probably failing to identify the real causes of "distress" in your home or office (and hence are not dealing with them). Stress is a natural part of life—smoking is not! The general adaptation syndrome guarantees the survival of the species—cigarette, pipe, and cigar smoking do not! Smoking stimulates your circulatory and nervous systems, which increases your heart rate, blood pressure, blood sugar levels, and general cardiac output. In essence, you are turning inward by stimulating your system and trying to protect yourself against the outside stimulus. Your body needs to be in good working order to cope with the stresses of everyday life. Smoking directly limits your body's ability to do this. The guilt and shame that accompany addiction to nicotine lead to a vicious cycle: the very cigarette you light up to cope with stress then becomes another stress in your life!

Coping with stress affects eating behavior as well. During the stress response the body stops digesting food as it prepares for fight or flight. Nothing can lead to a postmeal disaster as readily as being uptight while eating. Ever eat a really fine meal and wonder why you have a stomachache, headache, or just feel in a lousy mood? The answer, in a word, is stress. If you are going to lunch with the boss and you're really nervous, eat lightly. If possible get the business dispensed with before you start eating. Ever notice that in the movies real emotional upheaval in a restaurant scene is portrayed as an uneaten meal? So when uptight eat light or even skip a meal.

Stopping Smoking

Thirty million Americans have given up cigarette smoking. Another 55 million Americans are involved in physical exercise. The nation is into fitness and health. Some corporations are providing incentives and educational programs for their employees to encourage a healthy approach to living. More and more, people who indulge in addictive behaviors like smoking are being viewed in a negative light by superiors, peers, and subordinates in the work setting. Those who persist in smoking are viewed with greatly reduced esteem and may find themselves operating in reduced corridors of power and decision making. People will not sit next to you, may fail to invite you to certain meetings, will stand away from you during a conversation, and will generally begin subtle or overt forms of avoidance of you and your office. Worst of all, your superiors may view you as an example of poor health and lacking in self-control. You may be skipped over when it's time for promotions, and a healthier, better-controlled man or woman may move ahead of you. One way to find out how dependent you are on smoking at work is to see how uncomfortable you become when forced to abstain.

Here are some suggestions for quitting successfully.

- Most people do it on their own. Don't be afraid to try—even if you have to try many times. Every cigarette you don't smoke contributes to your health. It takes years for a smoker to catch up with a nonsmoker in terms of the reduced incidence of diseases like lung cancer.
- Consciously cut down on the amount you smoke each day until you reach zero. Not everyone can do it cold turkey. Tapering off slowly will make withdrawal a little easier. You can increase the time interval between cigarettes and the amount of time it takes to smoke a single cigarette—this will automatically reduce the number of cigarettes consumed in a single day. Keep a written record on a small card you can place in the cellophane liner of your cigarette pack. Remember, you are heading for zero!
- Try quitting with a partner. This need not be a spouse. Pair up with another smoker and support each other's commitment to stop completely. Call each other on the phone if you feel the urge to light up—even in the middle of the night. This is the approach called "phone therapy" developed by Alcoholics Anonymous, and it works for many people.
- Smoking behavior is often cued by certain internal states, external events, places, or people. Become familiar with the cues that trigger your smoking behavior. Avoid those that you can and stay mentally vigilant in the face of those that are unavoidable. Anticipate them and use phone therapy if needed.
- Try keeping dead butts in a jar with a little water in it. Visualizing and smelling what tobacco is really about will help to turn off the habit. Inhale some smoke and then blow it through a clean tissue. This is what is going into your lungs!
- For oral types, chew sugarless gum or munch on toothpicks.
- If you need to keep your hands busy, get some worry beads.

132

- Find more direct ways to deal with stress; get into stress avoidance and stress coping at the source of the problem.
- If you find you can't manage quitting on your own, join a mutual support program. You will be among kindred souls who will help reinforce your desire to quit.

WHICH APPETITES ARE WE FEEDING?

Eating behavior can be of a compulsive nature just as drug consumption often is. Immediately some of you may say, "So what! Let people who like to eat enjoy themselves. Does it really matter if we put on a few extra pounds? Everyone can't look like a fashion model! We need some 'love handles' to grab on to. I like my men [women] on the big side!"

Obesity and its associated health risks can't be sloughed off. Those who are overweight are prone to a wide variety of illnesses, including high blood pressure with its attendant risks of stroke and heart attack. The heart attack risk is enhanced by high levels of blood cholesterol and fat and low levels of the protective high-density-lipoprotein (HDL) cholesterol. Obese people are at greater risk of diabetes, certain forms of cancer, gallstones, arthritis, venous thrombosis, chronic bronchitis, accidents including those which are fatal, and surgical complications. And if the people in your company who make decisions about hiring, firing, raises, and promotions look askance at obesity, the results can hurt your career and your income. Although Americans generally have been getting fatter over the last eighty years, people are actually eating less and getting fewer calories than they did in 1900. The explanation is in the change in activity levels. Our modern technological advances have drastically reduced the amount of physical exercise we get. We walk less, lift less; in fact, we do everything less except sit. When we were more physically active we ate more to keep up our energy stores. So now we eat less, but the severe decline in physical exercise has allowed that amount of food we do not burn to turn into fat.

The ideal is regular exercise and a diet that cuts down on

the quantity of food consumed without lessening too much the intake of required nutrients. The best way to lose weight is to adopt a pattern of eating that maintains balanced nutrition while reducing calorie intake sensibly. If any of the fad diets really worked over the long haul, there would be no need for new ones! In my local paper the other night there were six ads for "diet centers." One is the biggest, one is the oldest, one guarantees no pills, another no dangerous diets, and all have testimonials with "before and after" photographs.

Every year millions of pounds are shed and every year the same millions of pounds are put back on. The basic problem seems to be that we want someone else to do it for us. We want instant magic—instant long-lasting magic. What is really required is a basic change in patterns of eating. While diets of all kinds may have a temporary effect, permanent changes in eating habits are the key to long-range success. This means the burden of responsibility falls right back into our own laps. And that is exactly where it belongs. The true bottom line on the issue of obesity is that we must reassume the responsibility for our own lifestyles. If you are concerned about your weight, then recognize that you can do something about it. You have to want to, and you have to face the fact that your eating behavior may resemble a chemical addiction. How? Addiction can be defined as (1) compulsion, followed by (2) negative consequences and (3) loss of control. This is why I am stressing regaining control over your own lifestyle and eating behavior. Too busy making a living to work into an active exercise routine? Did you ever stop to think that your acquisitive years may be cut short by what you are *not* doing *now?*

A pound of fat is the equivalent of about 3,500 calories. A surplus of just 100 calories a day will turn into ten pounds in a year. A brisk twenty-minute walk will use up these same calories. Look at it this way: every time you eat 3,500 calories less than you expend, you use up a pound of fatty tissue. A deficit of 500 calories a day (eating 2,000 and using up 2,500) will lead to a loss of one pound a week (that adds up to fifty-two pounds a year).

For many adults, eating has become the classic example of "looking for the right thing in the wrong place." If being fed in the earliest stages of life is associated with alleviation of hunger, the receiving of love and affection, and a sense of everything being right with the world, then it is easy to see how eating serves the same functions for the adult. However, eating can only *symbolize* these other forms of gratification. Food cannot replace love. Eating oneself through loneliness or anxiety does not address the root of the problem. Yes, it is a primitive method for returning to a better emotional state, but it is a most indirect route for having the other needs met. This type of eating is symbolic pleasure and always leaves one "hungry." Frustrated people who overeat only amplify the frustration, which leads to more eating, which leads to obesity. It can become a vicious cycle. It should be clear by now that whatever model you use to examine the phenomenon (analytic or behavioral), eating has come to mean many things in our society. Food acts as a tranquilizer for some people; it is a reward for others; while many just hurry through meals as if they are nothing more than a necessary nuisance. Once you stop and examine what role—other than plain survival—eating plays in your life, you can begin to make the necessary changes in your eating behavior. Some recent research at UCLA indicates that eating the right nutrients but drastically reduced calories may increase the human life span.

Nutritionists counsel us to eat a healthful breakfast that will fuel us for a morning's work, then a small lunch and a small dinner. The majority of Americans have sedentary jobs. Our bodies do not require the kind of refueling (in terms of calories) that our ancestors needed in 1900 for a job like lumberjacking. We seem to have this mental set which says that if we put in a hard day's work at the office we deserve to eat a "hearty" meal. If we skip breakfast and eat large lunches as well, we are headed for a caloric disaster and our waistlines will show it.

Watch out for food additives too. They can alter mood as quickly as any other drug. Additives are used to color food, lengthen shelf life, enhance taste, and make food look more attractive. Even dog food is manufactured to look appealing to the human eye. Additives are non-nutrient chemicals, most of which are innocuous. There are some 2,800 substances which are intentionally added to the foods we eat. Some additives like red dye #2 or DDT are dangerous. Two food additives are worthy of special mention because they figure so prominently in the American diet: salt and sugar.

Both sugar and salt are added in voluminous amounts to a wide variety of foodstuffs. We know they can be found in such items as sweetened cereals and pretzels. But have you checked the labels of other food items, such as the salt content in tomato juice or soup or bread, or the sugar in granola or ketchup or peanut butter? These are the "hidden" food additives. The average American eats around 128 pounds of sugar a year, which makes sugar our leading food additive. Salt comes in second; Americans eat an average of 15 pounds of salt a year. That comes to about 3 teaspoons of salt a day, far more than our body requires to stay healthy. Both sugar and salt tastes are acquired and are,

Problems Associated With:

Sugar	Salt
Tooth decay: worst when sweets are consumed between meals.	*Hypertension* (high blood pressure): salt is believed to be the main precipitant.
Obesity: sugar adds to the intake of more calories than we use up, which turn into fat.	*Kidney disease:* continuous dumping of excess sodium can lead to kidney malfunction.
Aggravates diabetes: obesity is the highest risk factor for diabetics; they must restrict their overall calories and sugar intake.	*Edema:* excess sodium can increase water in and around body tissues, leading to swelling. Figures in premenstrual tension.
Heart disease: sugar contributes to risk because it releases insulin, which directs the conversion of blood glucose into fatty acids and triglycerides, which promote the development of atherosclerosis.	*Heart disease and stroke:* excess sodium increases likelihood of both.

therefore, subject to change once we decide to do so. Listed below are some hints on how to change salt and sugar eating habits.

Sugar	Salt
Do your own baking and cut down on the amount of sugar you use.	Study food package ingredients carefully.
Don't reward kids or adults with sweets.	Cut out soft drinks with salt added. Switch from club soda to plain seltzer.
Cut out soft drinks. This change alone can bring about a 50% reduction in your sugar intake.	Be on the lookout for high-sodium vegetables like grits, spinach, and sauerkraut.
Reduce sugar in coffee and tea.	Don't add any salt at the dinner table.
Serve fruit. Fresh is best. If you use canned or frozen, look for those packed in water instead of sweet syrup.	Gradually cut back on the amount of salt you are already using.
Eat unsugared cereals for breakfast.	Try other herbs, condiments, and spices.
Stop buying candy or other sweets for the home or office.	Purchase a low-salt cookbook.
Study ingredients on package labels carefully.	Look for foods marked "low-salt" or "low-sodium" when you shop.
Don't use sweets for an energy lift—only diabetics benefit from this. The lift lasts only minutes for the rest of us.	Avoid fast-food restaurants—they use a lot of salt.
	Cut down on processed foods—you will avoid salt and many other additives. Buy fresh food whenever possible

Diet can have both subtle and dramatic effects on our mood and behavior. Consider the following examples:

- Dr. Richard Wurtman of MIT states, "It's likely that early in life people make associations between the consumption of certain foods and changes in how they feel. Then, later on, they unconsciously turn to these foods to re-create the desired feelings."

• The eating of sugars and starches (carbohydrates) can raise the level of a brain chemical called serotonin. Serotonin is associated with feeling relaxed, calm, sleepy, less depressed, and less sensitive to pain. According to Dr. Judith Wurtman of MIT, this may be the reason why so many people binge on carbohydrates when feeling anxious or depressed. She states, "It may also explain why high-protein, low-carbohydrate weight-reduction diets usually fail. These diets cause a serotonin deficiency in the brain which in turn could trigger carbohydrate craving to correct the imbalance."

• Neurotransmitters are brain chemicals that transmit messages between nerve cells. Certain nutrients alter brain levels of these chemicals that regulate a wide variety of brain functions and have a direct effect on mood and performance. One example of such a nutrient is tryptophan, an amino acid found in protein foods like meat, chicken, and fish. Eating such foods raises blood levels of tryptophan, which causes increases in brain levels of serotonin.

• Similarly, another amino acid from protein foods called tyrosine is associated with increased levels of another neurotransmitter called norepinephrine. Norepinephrine and serotonin are viewed by psychiatry as playing major roles in mental depression. Nearly all psychiatric drugs used to treat depression increase brain transmission by one or both of these chemicals.

• Dr. Judith Rapoport of the National Institute of Mental Health reports that children who are high consumers of caffeine (in soft drinks and iced tea) were described as more nervous, more hyperactive, and more easily frustrated and angered than were children who typically consumed less caffeine. She also reported that, contrary to popular impression, sugar had a calming effect on the children in her study. This finding is consistent with the known effects of carbohydrates on serotonin levels in the brain.

As more is learned about the effects of many nutrients on human behavior we will be better able to control our own mood and performance through dietary means. This could ultimately mean less introduction of manufactured drugs into our systems and the return to more natural forms of "self-medication." These studies bring new meaning to the notion "You are what you eat."

Some Hints for Eating Right at Work

- Start with a good breakfast. It will help you be more efficient in the mornings and help you eat smaller lunches.
- Coffee and tea during the workday are fine as long as you don't experience caffeinism. You may want to intersperse fruit juices and other beverages.
- Large business lunches can make you feel stuffed and lethargic and make it difficult to get back to work. Light lunches are good for health and business.
- Alcoholic drinks have "empty" calories and can alter your mood, motor coordination, and ability to think clearly. Go easy on booze, especially at business lunches. People tend to play follow-the-leader with alcohol. Decide what you will do before you get to the restaurant.
- Do not depend on sweets for "instant energy." The lift is elusive. Try a piece of fresh fruit, which contains fructose, a sugar that has fewer calories.
- If you need something in your mouth, try sugarless gum.
- When dining out with customers, pick a restaurant that is not noisy or crowded. The setting is as important as the food in terms of pleasure and digestion.
- Rich desserts are hard to resist. But why spoil a nice meal with a lot of guilt and empty calories? Don't say yes when you want to say no.

- Get out for lunch. Don't make a habit of eating at your desk. Take a break from the work routine. Celebrate your lunch hour. Try to take a walk after eating. Let lunch be a total experience, not just a break from working.
- Bad news and food don't mix. Reading about tragedy in the daily paper while eating is not a good idea. Remember when the Vietnam war poured out of TV sets during dinner? It's an unhealthy combination (stress again).
- Don't wolf down your food. The antacid manufacturers are already making a fortune.
- When you've had a good day, reward yourself with a nutritious and tasty meal, not a big one.
- Plan enough time for meals during the workday.
- If you eat at your desk often enough, just sitting at your desk can become a cue to eat.
- If a busy schedule or deadline necessitates eating while you work, eat lightly, avoid spicy foods, have light snacks handy, and go easy on caffeine.

Common sense can allow you to enjoy the pleasures of eating without the guilt that interferes. Recognize the central role that food and eating play in your life. Then keep the ideal in mind: regular exercise and a diet that cuts down on quantity without sacrificing nutrition.

DRUGS AND SPORTS

In 1982 reports of widespread use of cocaine in the National Football League made front-page news in the *New York Times* and in *Sports Illustrated* magazine. Don Reese, a former defensive lineman with several NFL teams, made the following claim on the cover page of *Sports Illustrated:*[5]

Cocaine can be found in quantity throughout the NFL. It's pushed on players, often from the edge of the practice field.

Sometimes it's pushed by players. Prominent players. Just as it controlled me, it now controls and corrupts the game, because so many players are on it. To ignore this fact is to be short-sighted and stupid.

Other famous players have admitted to the use of this drug. There have been reports of cocaine use by players of other professional sports including baseball, basketball, and boxing. Estimates of the actual incidence of drugs in professional sports are hard to come by. Like other aspects of the drug scene, it depends on whom you are speaking with. The media tend to hype this kind of sensational phenomenon, and sports management tends to cover it up or play it down. The players with a drug problem are the ones who suffer. But they aren't the only ones. Entire teams, players' families, the good name of a school, the reputation of coaches—all are casualties of the athletic drug wars. And the problem is not restricted to professional or even college sports. Competitive athletics start in the junior-high-school or middle-school years, and this is where we must focus our attention to understand the roots of the multiple relationship between sports and drugs.

Leo Durocher said it many years ago: "Nice guys finish last!" The name of the game in competitive athletics is winning. Sometimes that means winning at all costs. The costs are most often paid by the athletes themselves. There are many diet and exercise regimens used for building the powerful bodies that are required in many sports—most notably weight lifting, wrestling, boxing, football and most other contact sports. The enhancement of regular nutrition may start with megadoses of vitamins (which remain unproven in developing athletic prowess). Powerful drugs like anabolic steroids are sometimes used to develop large muscles. Soviet-bloc athletes have been challenged a number of times during world Olympic meets as to their use of such drugs in body building. Even some female athletes use them, and have also been known to take male hormones in an effort to build bulk. The use of hormones and steroids can be very dangerous and involves a whole host of side effects and adverse reactions, which is why most coaches and sports-medicine professionals shun them.

A variety of anesthetic and analgesic drugs are used in sports. These are the chemicals that deaden the sensation of pain and allow injured players to return to the playing field. Some are short acting and are applied topically, like Lidocaine. Others are longer acting and are taken internally, like Demerol. The hotter the competition and the more that is riding on the outcome of a game, the more likely it is that these drugs will be used to keep the better players on the field. Pain is a symptom of an injury or trauma and helps in the diagnosis of such problems. When pain is masked, the player is not aware of the extent or seriousness of the injury. And in sports like football, you go out and play even if you are in pain. Winning is everything and the player is supposed to bear pain like a "real man." But in the eighth grade, at age thirteen or fourteen? It's hard to sit on the bench when family, friends, and schoolmates are cheering your team on. So sometimes the players themselves ask for the drugs so they can get back into the action. And sometimes coaches push the kids to take the drugs. And the parents either ignore or deny the whole thing.

Another facet of drugs and sports is the social side. The reward for many athletes, including the younger ones, after a game well played (or even not so well played) is often a drug. Whether it's a surreptitious can of beer or a marijuana joint or a snort of cocaine, many young athletes look forward to getting high after the big game or meet. Certainly this is not true of all school-age athletes, some of whom shun drugs in any form as part of their caring for their bodies. But it's awfully hard to resist peer-group pressure in a setting where being one of the boys or girls is all-important. It's easy to see how quickly the use of pleasure drugs can spread within a tightly knit social group like an athletic team. Coaches have very little influence against this kind of pressure. Beer drinking in particular is seen as cute and part of the macho trip, so parents tend to make light of such drug use. It is not uncommon these days for girls who want to get closer to athletes socially to use drugs to attract them. This is a game played with a vengeance at the college and professional level, but it begins much earlier. More and more parents are beginning to ask where the team and the cheerleaders are, late on a Saturday night, and why it is so hard for these kids to get up on Sunday mornings. Could be they are hung over. Losers get high too— it's called relief drinking (winning is called celebration drinking).

When I attended a Big Ten college in the midwest in 1960, I roomed with a second-string fullback on the football team. He took me to several team parties and I have never seen such heavy drinking in my life—replete with drunkenness, fights, sexual antics, throwing up, chugalug contests, and drag racing. The ethic was "play hard–party hard" and never miss a practice (no matter how rotten you feel). Looking back, I now recognize some of these high-spirited antics as alcoholic drinking by at least several of the team members. My roommate summed up the whole thing very succinctly: "You practice hard all week, do whatever you're told by the coaches, kick ass and play your heart out on Saturday afternoon and then . . . drink, screw and raise holy hell on Saturday night!"

But he also opened my eyes to something else. Some of the guys were taking some "pep" pills to get up for the big game. The pills, otherwise known as amphetamines, create the feeling of tremendous physical and mental prowess. There were several "speed" scandals in professional football during the 1960s and '70s. Cocaine serves the same function. These stimulant drugs create a powerful elevation of mood, extreme euphoria, and feelings of power and grandeur. One of the things about many sports events that attracts young athletes is that they can find a natural high on the playing field. Some learn to use stimulant drugs to intensify these feelings. Others look for the drugs to duplicate this same exhilaration off the playing field. Once it gets to the point of regular drug use, like daily snorting of cocaine or freebasing (smoking the pure essence of cocaine), the drug takes over and the athletics go right down the tube. Some wealthy pro athletes have lost their fortunes and their playing ability because of drugs like cocaine.

HEALTH PROMOTION IN THE WORKPLACE

My drinking got out of hand to the point where it was interfering with my job. I was missing deadlines, missing important meetings, and calling in sick a lot. It took a couple of years for this to happen, and when it got bad enough my supervisor called me in and told me to shape up or ship out. He also told me about the company psychologist whom I could go see in confidence. At first I thought he was off the wall. Why would I want to talk to a "shrink"? I wasn't crazy. But I was so afraid of losing my job that I went anyway. He helped me to see that the bulk of my problems stemmed from my inability to handle alcohol. He sent me to A.A. and a therapist. I have been sober for just over a year now. My job and my marriage have both improved since I stopped drinking. Thank goodness my company had an employee assistance program or I would have been out of work and out of luck.

—INSURANCE SALESMAN

Too often people talk about the world of work and the private life of a person as if they were totally separate realities. Certainly there are profound differences, but the essential person remains unchanged in both settings. The problems that affect someone at home are carried into the workplace just as work-related problems are often brought into the home. Most wives can tell what kind of day their husbands have had at work by just looking at their faces when they come through the door. The whole range of human problems and ills have a direct impact upon the work site. Divorces, marital squabbles, problems with kids, poor health, financial troubles, drug abuse, spouse abuse, alcohol abuse and alcoholism, sexual dysfunction—all have a way of eroding productivity and efficiency at work. Over 20 million people—15 percent of the American population—need mental-health services at any time, according to the President's Commission on Mental Health, and 25 percent of the population "is under the kind of emotional stress that results in symptoms of depression and anxi-

144

ety." Most of these people work, and when they arrive at the office or plant their problems arrive with them. The impact of alcoholism alone is staggering. Drug misuse and abuse account for an untold percentage of problems as well.

More than 400 companies have set up preventive programs for their employees over the past decade. These companies must feel that one way or another they will pay for employees' mental

Company	Type of Program
Hospital Corporation of America	Pays its employees by the mile for staying healthy by swimming, jogging, or cycling.
Dow Chemical Company (Texas Division)	Pays cash incentives for their employees to stop smoking.
Mendocino County (California) Office of Education	Cash credit is offered to employees who file medical claims of less than $500 in a year.
New York Telephone Company	A staff of 40 physicians, covering 80,000 employees in more than 1,000 locations. Boasts a 90% success rate in treating hypertension; offers courses in smoking cessation, stress and hypertension control.
International Business Machines	Offers voluntary health screening exam, which has revealed more than 322,000 health problems in 13 years (35% of them previously unknown).
Kimberly-Clark Corporation	Employees fill out a 40-page medical history, submit to a battery of lab tests, and run through a treadmill exercise test during which their heart rate is monitored. Has an EAP and a $2.5 million fitness facility.
Pepsico, Inc.	Maintains a fitness center with a full-time director. Top management has a separate facility. Center can monitor via a computer the amount of calories burned by an employee over a week's time.

and physical problems. Linda B. Nielson, Director of Counseling Services for Insight, the employee assistance program (EAP) at the Kennecott Corporation's Utah Copper Division, says of companies: "They may pay in supervisory time spent trying to improve job performance, or in exorbitant medical costs, or the costs of absenteeism and turnover. Or they can pay for preventive services like Insight."

In New York State in 1982 only 12 percent of the work force had access to an EAP. Listed above are some examples of company "wellness" programs.[6] These companies and others like them have taken the position that problems such as alcoholism, drug addiction, smoking, overuse of sugar and salt, and poor dental hygiene are preventable.

The lever of the job is what makes EAPs successful. You may not want to admit you are crazy or that you have a drinking or drugging problem, but the last thing you want to do is lose

---

How to Recognize a Good Employee Assistance Program

- Program is well advertised, so that all levels of management and labor know about it and how to use it.
- Supervisors are trained to make referrals to the program.
- Employees can gain access to the EAP counselor in privacy, and all communications are held in the strictest confidence.
- Corporate health benefits provide coverage for physical and mental problems, including alcohol and drug abuse.
- EAP counselor has a good list of resources for services for which the benefit package provides coverage.
- Referrals include self-help groups like Alcoholics Anonymous and women's support groups as well as professional practitioners.
- Benefit package includes both in-patient and out-patient treatment of chemical dependencies.
- Supervisors need never know the nature of the personal problem. Their only concern is job-related functioning by the worker.

your job. Besides the financial aspect, Americans have a lot of self-esteem tied up in their work. The pressure of the EAP is strictly job-related, but by getting the employee (and in some cases employer) to proper diagnosis and needed treatment, the whole man or woman benefits right along with the company.

YOU AND DRUGS AT WORK— A SELF-RATING QUESTIONNAIRE

Take a few minutes to fill out this questionnaire as honestly as possible. Place a check mark next to the alternative that best answers the question.

It's hard enough getting through the average workday. If you find that you are balancing a drug act along with your work responsibilities, you are walking a thin line toward disaster. Whatever your reasons for using drugs at work, you will want to exercise some real caution. Remember the three hallmarks of addiction: (1) a compulsion to use the drug, (2) negative consequences due to use of the drug, and (3) loss of control over the drug (and your life). The damage done by alcohol, caffeine, nicotine, and overeating are far more subtle than the drugs we perceive as more overt tools of abuse. But they take their toll over time, eroding the quality of our lives at work and at home. You are in charge of what goes into your body.

Often	Some-times	Seldom	Never	
_____	_____	_____	_____	1. Do you drink more than 5 cups of coffee during a workday?
_____	_____	_____	_____	2. Do you use pleasure drugs during working hours?

147

Often	Some-times	Seldom	Never	
——	——	——	——	3. Do you feel that drugs help you to work better?
——	——	——	——	4. Do you smoke cigarettes at work?
——	——	——	——	5. Is alcohol a part of your business lunches?
——	——	——	——	6. Do you depend on food with a lot of sugar to give you a lift at work?
——	——	——	——	7. Do you take tranquilizers to deal with the stress of your job?
——	——	——	——	8. Do any drugs that you take interfere with your ability to do your job?
——	——	——	——	9. Has anyone at work ever talked to you about your drinking or drug taking?
——	——	——	——	10. Do you miss work because of drug or alcohol use?
——	——	——	——	11. Are you late or do you leave early because of drug or alcohol use?
——	——	——	——	12. Do people at work hassle you about your smoking?

DRUGS AND THE WORKPLACE

Often	Some- times	Seldon	Never	
_____	_____	_____	_____	13. Is your job so boring that you need to get high just to get through the day?
_____	_____	_____	_____	14. Do you ever drink or drug before going to work?
_____	_____	_____	_____	15. Have drugs ever interfered with memory function at work?
_____	_____	_____	_____	16. Do you arrange your workday around your drug taking?

How to score: 3 points for every "often" response
2 points for every "occasionally" response
1 point for every "seldom" response
0 points for every "never" response

0–16: Zero indicates no problem at all. The closer you get to 16, the more you must start thinking about how drugs affect you at work.

17–32: Yellow Alert. Drugs are too much a part of your work life and perhaps your private life as well. Cut down and be careful.

33–48: Red Alert. You are in real trouble. It's time to seek professional help for your drug problem!

CHAPTER FOUR

Drugs as Medicine

People have been searching for relief from pain and suffering for thousands of years. The practice of modern medicine is an art that draws upon many sciences, including pharmacology. Our ancestors explored the flora and fauna in their environment for aids to health as well as relief from pain. The technological explosion of the last hundred years has yielded new medicines and a whole health-care industry. By 1981 the total expense for health care in America had reached 9.8 percent of the gross national product (that's more than $162 billion). As a nation we spend billions each year on the ethical, or prescription, medicines prescribed for us by our doctors and even more billions for nonprescription, or over-the-counter, medications that allow us to "doctor" ourselves.

The medications that we take have a profound effect on our physical, mental, emotional, spiritual, and social selves, although we tend to restrict our thinking about medicine to the purely physical. The blossoming of the concepts of holistic medicine, which germinated with the South African philosopher and statesman Jan Christiaan Smuts in the 1920s, has allowed us to see ourselves as whole persons and not simply the sum of our parts (organs). What we eat, how we live, the quality of our environment, our own health practices or lack of same, are all taken into consideration when considering our state of health. The very term "health" is no longer applied solely to its complement, illness and disease; it now relates to positive practices and feeling good. The use and abuse of drugs as medicine are part and parcel of the concerns of holistic medicine, and as such deserve our serious attention. The time has come for us to assume full responsibility for what we put into our bodies in the name of health and not abdicate that responsibility to others.

YOU AND YOUR DOCTOR

Illness and disease are frightening realities. Children take their cues from adults regarding their attitudes toward being sick, getting well, being well, suffering and enduring pain, taking medicine, and relating to doctors and other health-care professionals. One of the first rude awakenings for children, who tend to see parents as all-knowing and omnipotent, is that parents must often turn to "strangers" (family doctors or pediatricians) for help in alleviating illness and discomfort. How we perceive, talk about, and relate to doctors gives a very powerful message to our children. If adults react to the doctor as a source of good counsel and healthful medicine, then the child will tend to trust and listen to the doctor. If, on the other hand, the doctor and the medicine are viewed with suspicion and caution, then our child will pick up these attitudes. If our children see us caring for our own bodies and thereby acting as partners in health with our doctors, they get one kind of message. If they see us not caring for ourselves and waiting for our bodies to break down so we can take them to a technician (doctor) for repair, much like our automobiles, they get an entirely different message.

Consider how you do, in fact, relate to your doctor(s). Take a few moments to fill out the questionnaire below. Check off either "true" or "false" for each item and answer as honestly as you can.

True   False

1. When my doctor uses terms I do not understand I ask for a simpler explanation.

2. Upon arriving home, if I'm not sure about something my doctor said in the office, I will call and ask questions.

3. I have a right, as a patient, to ask as many questions as I need to.

4. If my doctor gives me written instructions and I can't read the handwriting, I ask to have it written more clearly.

5. If I must wait a long time (more than 15 minutes) to see the doctor I will mention this to him or her.

6. I do not hesitate to ask my doctor about medications prescribed for me (side effects, dosage, interactions, etc.).

7. I make suggestions to my doctor concerning my health.

8. I make sure to tell my doctor about any drugs I am taking (including illicit drugs).

9. If I feel a second opinion is in order, I will tell this to my doctor.

10. I consider myself an equal partner with my doctor when it comes to caring for my health.

11. I will ask my doctor to prescribe generic drugs instead of name brands.

12. If the doctor indicates a course of medical or surgical treatment, I ask questions about risks versus benefits.

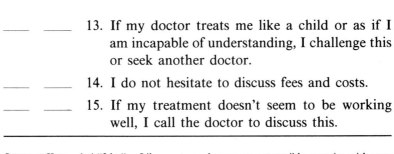

True   False

             13. If my doctor treats me like a child or as if I am incapable of understanding, I challenge this or seek another doctor.

             14. I do not hesitate to discuss fees and costs.

             15. If my treatment doesn't seem to be working well, I call the doctor to discuss this.

SCORING KEY: 1–4 "false": Like most people, you are not terribly assertive with your doctor.

5–9 "false": You are taking too much for granted and not sharing in your own health care.

10 or more "false": You are reacting like a child to your doctor and have totally placed your health in someone else's hands.

People seem to need to "look good" in front of their doctors; we don't want physicians to look down on us. Yet it is terribly important that we report accurately and unashamedly anything affecting our health status. Denial of drug use is one of the things people get caught up in with doctors. Part of this denial may be outright manipulation, but more often it is a psychological phenomenon called "transference." The patient automatically and unconsciously generalizes and "transfers" from past interpersonal relationships with authority figures (doctors are certainly authority figures in our society). We tend to carry over feelings and needs about our parents to our doctors. We act like children in front of them, almost as if they were our own parents. When you combine this transference with the wish we have to see doctors as omnipotent and infallible, you can get some idea about what is going on, emotionally, when you visit your doctor.

Doctors are aware of this "godlike" pedestal that patients put them on. When they are treated this way they go right along with it because it's easier. They have to answer fewer questions that challenge their expertise, and they don't have to spend as much time working hard to explain medical terminology in terms the lay person can understand. This explains, in part, why some doctors have such large practices. Visits can be kept brief when we fail to actively exercise our responsibility as a partner in the relationship.

Dr. Thomas Preston in his book *The Clay Pedestal* suggests we re-examine the doctor-patient relationship:[1]

> The notion of the consummate physician helping the distressed patient during his or her hour of need is undoubtedly the most enduring attraction for the public in its view of the medical profession. The myth of the selfless physician marshalling the forces of science for the welfare of his patients, however, has come to conceal reality rather than to reflect it, and to deflect inquiry into the true nature of medical practice, which falls far short of this mythical ideal.

Dr. Preston points out that frequently the most serious and consequential criticisms of modern medical practice come from the physicians themselves, working and speaking through conventional medical forums.

Educate your children so that they can learn about their own bodies and health issues. Help them learn to deal with health in its fullest sense—the promotion of good health habits and a sense of personal responsibility for that health. Don't let them think of health as important only when something is wrong. Here are some hints on how to accomplish this.

1. Encourage your children to learn the different parts of their bodies. Teach them correct anatomical names. Make a game of it. Use illustrations.
2. When preparing to visit a doctor be upbeat and positive. The child will pick up any negative vibrations that you give off.
3. When at the doctor's, encourage your child to ask questions about any aspect of his or her health or body.

Set the stage by rehearsing at home, and by asking the doctor a question yourself.

4. Don't shy away from "what if . . . ?" questions about health. If you don't know the answer, look it up, or write the question down and save it for your next visit to the doctor's office.
5. Don't talk about doctors as if they were infallible. Don't talk about medicines as if they were magic potions. Everyone makes mistakes, including doctors. Communicate confidence but not omnipotence regarding the doctor.
6. Don't make it sound as if all of life's ills or pains can be alleviated by medicine or medication.
7. Use real medical terms but define them. Cutesy-poo terms don't teach even if they do amuse.
8. When someone in the family is ill, kids see this as a serious matter. Don't shut them out. Explain things on a level they can understand. Let them help in small ways to make the sick person feel better.
9. Teach your child to care for his or her own health through positive modeling of dental care, accident prevention, not smoking, not abusing drugs, moderation in food and drink, and so on.
10. Realize that childhood is a time when lifelong attitudes and health behaviors are forming. Don't leave it to others to shape positive health habits and attitudes in your children.
11. Remember that kids are sharp. They have a built-in "crap detector." They know when you are lying to them or avoiding an issue. Be straight with them.

Tell it like it is, especially with young children. But don't feel compelled to tell them everything at once.

John is in the second grade. He comes home one afternoon and asks his mother, "Where do I come from?" His mother, wishing to be very contemporary and informative, launches into a fifteen-minute lecture on the birds and the bees (human style). After listening patiently to his mother's lecture on human sexuality, little John looks up at her and states, "Ralph in my class comes from Chicago. Where do I come from?"

It makes a lot of sense to allow the physicians, dentists, nurses, and other health-care professionals to act as educated guides and consultants to us regarding our health. It does not make any sense to allow them to take over and control it. The bottom line is that it is your body and you must ultimately pay for your healthy habits or lack of them. By forming a co-equal and active partnership with these health professionals you are using the best of both worlds: responsible self-care and guidance from your consultants. If you don't like or trust the advice from one consultant, find another. This is one area of your life where failing to be assertive can get you into serious trouble.

Now let's get more specific about the role you play concerning drugs and your relationship with your doctor. Here is a questionnaire to test your knowledge about your use of medications.

True   False

____   ____   1. I know the names of all the drugs I take (both generic and brand name).

____   ____   2. I always take the medication as prescribed (both the amount and frequency).

____   ____   3. I always finish taking the medication even if I feel better.

____   ____   4. I ask my doctor about side effects when he or she offers me medication.

____   ____   5. I ask my doctor about the main effects (therapeutic benefit) that I can expect from a medication that he or she is prescribing for me.

True   False

_____ _____ 6. I naturally assume that brand-name drugs work better.

_____ _____ 7. I always tell my doctor, dentist, anesthesiologist, surgeon, about any drugs I am taking (street, prescription, over-the-counter, alcohol).

_____ _____ 8. I always ask my doctor if the drug he or she is prescribing can interact with other drugs.

_____ _____ 9. I always ask if I should take my medication before or after eating.

_____ _____ 10. I would never give a friend one of my prescription medications or take one of his or hers.

_____ _____ 11. I always ask my doctor if I should restrict any of my activities when taking a medication.

_____ _____ 12. I take the drug advertising I see on television with a very large grain of salt.

_____ _____ 13. I always ask if it is okay to drink alcohol when taking a prescribed or OTC medication.

_____ _____ 14. I always ask my doctor to write down important drug-taking instructions or cautions.

_____ _____ 15. I always ask my doctor or pharmacist about the best way to store my medication.

SCORING KEY: 1–4 "false": You need to learn more about the medications you use and the way you use them.

5–9 "false": You are letting someone else take over your own health care. Better hope they have told you everything you need to know to avoid problems.

10 or more "false": You may have already taken drugs the wrong way and experienced unnecessary side effects or even adverse reactions. You need to regain control over your own body and health.

(Question 6 is the only one to which "false" is the correct answer.)

POSITIVE PRACTICES REGARDING THE USE OF MEDICATIONS

Know what you are taking. Some drugs have very similar-sounding names but are dramatically different in their uses and chemical action. For example, *Orinase* (tolbutamide) is a drug used to correct insulin deficiency, while *Ornade* (main ingredient, phenylpropanolamine) is a drug used for the relief of congestion of the nose, sinuses, and throat.

Have your doctor write down both the generic and the brand names (in legible writing). The generic name, or common name, refers to the active drug ingredient. The brand name is what the drug manufacturer chooses to call its product. For example, when we refer to the tranquilizer as Valium, we are using the brand name; the generic name for this drug is diazepam. In Canada, diazepam is marketed under no fewer than eleven different brand names. A four-state, four-year study released in 1982 by the National Center for Health Services Research revealed that pharmacists are virtually ignoring laws permitting the substitution of less expensive generic formulations. The percentage of substituting generic for brand name drugs was low: 8.6 percent in Vermont, 7.4 percent in Michigan, 5.1 percent in Wisconsin, and 2.6 percent in Rhode Island. Dr. Theodore Goldberg of Wayne State University Medical School, the study director, states: "Although the potential for substitution appears great in each state studied, the actual experience has been disappointing." The American Pharmaceutical Association points out that pharmacists lack financial incentives for dispensing generic drugs and that simplification of state laws together with increased experience by pharmacists in handling generics should lead to a substantial increase over the next five to ten years. All drug sales are increasing at 12 percent annually, but the generic market is moving ahead at 14 percent, according to the Generic Pharmaceutical Association. You should ask both your physician and pharmacist for generic equivalent drugs. You stand to save 25 percent or an average of $1.25 for each prescription.

It is a good idea to keep medicines in their original containers and to take these with you when traveling. In case of an overdose or other adverse reaction, the drug can be quickly identified—this could save your life! It might also be a good idea to purchase a book which contains color illustrations of common prescription pills to help you to identify yours by their color and other markings. Always read the label before taking medicine or you are liable to take the wrong stuff or the wrong dose.

Know why you are taking it. We have all heard so much about side effects that we often fail to focus on the positive reasons for taking a drug. It is vital that you tell your doctor everything that is bothering you so he or she can suggest the best course

Drug Factors[2]	Patient Factors	Physician Factors
dose levels	sex, age	training
multiple effects	body size and weight	diagnostic skill
absorption rate	pregnancy, nursing	therapeutic skill
distribution	pharmacogenetic fac-	experience with
metabolism	tors	drugs
excretion	biochemical status	concomitant therapy
duration	nutritional status	attitude toward drug
route of administra-	drug metabolism	therapy
tion	disease (vast multi-	attitude toward pa-
habituation	plicity of factors)	tient
addiction potential	idiosyncrasy, hyper-	attitude toward dis-
tolerance	sensitivity	ease
side effects	contraindications	
toxicity	precautions	
idiosyncratic reaction	toxicity	
hypersensitivity	margin of safety	
margin of safety	concomitant therapy	
precautions	personality factors	
contraindications	attitude toward dis-	
pharmaceutical prop-	ease, drugs, doc-	
erties	tors	
chemical properties	cost	
drug interactions		

of treatment. If that treatment includes medication, you should know specifically why that particular drug is recommended and what its benefits are. All drugs have what are called multiple actions. You want to know what the principal beneficial action is. You will also want to know about the other actions commonly referred to as side effects. The drug your doctor prescribes should be the "drug of best choice." Many factors go into this decision.

You will want to know if this drug is the best available for your illness or disease. You will want to know if the intended therapeutic actions outweigh any side effects or possible adverse reactions. Do not agree to any course of drug therapy until you thoroughly understand this benefit/risk ratio, the financial commitment involved, and have had all your questions answered. Do not permit any doctor to rush you through a discussion of the medications, as this is the part of your treatment you are in charge of at home.

Take only as prescribed. Some people like to alter dosages and intervals between dosages. "If one is good, two is better" can be just as dangerous as "I feel better so I'll only take half as much." Taking too little of a medication can put insufficient amounts of the drug into your body to bring about the desired therapeutic benefit. Overdosing or putting too much of a drug into your system can bring the drug to toxic (poisonous) levels in the body. People don't OD (overdose) only on drugs like heroin.

Make sure that you understand exactly how to take the drug. You must know the route of administration (oral, injection, topical, nasal, etc.), how often to take it (once a day, twice a day, etc.), what time of day to take it, whether to drink it down with water or something else, before or after mealtimes. Ask questions. Don't leave the doctor's office until you understand. Have the doctor write it out, or his nurse if you can't read his instructions.

Check with your doctor before modifying the amount or the frequency of your drug taking. If you should skip a dose, ask the doctor what to do—don't "double-up" on your own. Very often people stop taking their antibiotics as soon as they feel better. Symptoms may be responding to the medication, but the underlying illness causing these symptoms requires the full course of the medicine. Otherwise the symptoms may re-emerge. If your doctor told you to take the medicine for ten days, take it for the full ten days. Make sure you follow specific instructions given to you about any medication. Exceptions to this occur when there are side effects or adverse reactions (see below).

Dealing with side effects. As mentioned above, the taking of any drug is a delicate balance between risks and benefits. Here is an example. A person suffering the symptoms of a serious depression may be well advised to take a tricyclic antidepressive medication like Elavil (amitriptyline). Physicians and pharmacologists know that drugs like Elavil can significantly reduce (about 80 percent of the time) the depressive symptoms (loss of appetite, lack of energy, diminished interest in sex, sleep disturbance, feelings of hopelessness). They also know that certain side effects such as drowsiness, blurring of vision, dryness of the mouth, constipation, and impaired urination can be expected when this drug is taken. For most people the side effects become reduced over several weeks, but for others they may persist. In the case of the clinically depressed person the risks may be far outweighed by the benefits. The expected and unavoidable side effects may be seen as a small price to pay for a course of drug therapy designed to alleviate the debilitating effects of the depression. This kind of decision should be a joint venture between patient and doctor. If the precipitating events in the patient's environment can be identified, this will help in the treatment. In many cases psychotherapy may be indicated along with or instead of the medication. But if the depression proves unresponsive to talk therapy, the patient should not be denied drug therapy. After the patient has been on the medication for a while the doctor and patient can experiment by putting the patient on a "drug holiday" to see if the depressive symptoms return.

All drugs have multiple actions: the principal action (the benefit) and side effects. Make sure your doctor discusses both types of action when considering any drug therapy. This will help you to more intelligently weigh the risks and the benefits.

Dealing with adverse reactions. There are many patient factors involved in drug taking. Some people have idiosyncratic or hypersensitive reactions to drugs. Your doctor cannot usually predict these types of adverse reactions. The most extreme reactions are allergic in nature (ranging from a rash to anaphylactic shock). You must inform your doctor *immediately* if you suffer any adverse reaction. The doctor can change the dosage or switch to another medication. Remember, side effects can be predicted (and should be discussed with your doctor before taking the drug), but adverse reactions usually cannot. Ask your doctor before taking the drug if he is aware of any possible adverse reactions for that drug. Ask for the major warning symptoms of adverse reactions for that particular drug, or look in one of the many consumer guides to drugs. While it may seem like a good idea to cease taking a drug if you have an adverse reaction, the best thing you can do is speak to the doctor before the next scheduled dose. You should report all side effects, adverse reactions, and overdoses to the doctor. If you can't reach the doctor before your next scheduled dose, find out if he or she has another doctor "on call" and contact that doctor, or call your pharmacist, or contact a physician in the emergency room of a local hospital.

It is a good idea to keep a written record of all adverse reactions. You should note the names (generic and brand), dosage, and the actual reaction. It is important to know the generic name because another doctor might prescribe the same generic drug under a different brand name, which will lead to a repeat of the adverse reaction. Since most people use more than one doctor, it is important to become a full partner in your health-care record-keeping. You will want to keep a note on dosage because sometimes negative effects can be reduced by changing dose levels. You should inform your doctor of any known drug allergies— don't wait to be asked. It's also a good idea to wear a "medical alert" bracelet or necklace which states drug allergies. At the very least carry this information in your wallet (but don't bury it).

Informing the doctor about drugs you are taking. Most people are far too passive in the way they interact with their doctors. You must take responsibility for your end of the partnership. One way to do this is to tell your doctor about any other drugs you may have taken recently or plan to take again soon, as well as those you are presently taking. This includes any "street" or "recreational" drugs (marijuana, cocaine, ludes, amyl nitrate, etc.). Don't forget to include alcohol, nicotine, and caffeine as well. Be sure to tell your regular family doctor about any drugs prescribed by other physicians (even if they were prescribed some time ago, if you are liable to be using them the doctor must know about them). I have known former heroin addicts who were enrolled in methadone (a powerful synthetic narcotic) maintenance programs who did not tell their surgeons that they were on the program. So, naturally, the surgeon wrote a typical medication order for managing postoperative pain. Because these patients' bodies were regularly receiving 80 to 100 milligrams of methadone per day, the amount of postoperative analgesic (pain-killer) needed to successfully reduce pain was two to three times the normal dose. It always pays to level with the doctor, up front! After all, it's a confidential doctor-patient relationship. The only thing getting in your way is your image (your need to look "good" in front of your doctor). Be certain to tell not only your doctor but also your surgeon, anesthesiologist, and dentist about all the drugs you are taking. Again, don't forget to include street drugs and OTCs.

During pregnancy and breast feeding. Many drugs pass through the placenta and reach the fetus. Many also find their way into breast milk. In both these ways the drugs can be passed to the fetus or child. You must tell your doctor all the drugs you are taking as soon as you learn that you are pregnant. Now you have two lives to consider, and this dramatically alters the benefit-to-risk ratio. Therefore, a frank discussion with your gynecologist/obstetrition is in order to ensure both your health and that of your child. The same wisdom applies to the period when you are breast feeding.

The fetus is most sensitive to drugs during the first trimester (first twelve weeks) of pregnancy, so it's a good idea for women who *think* they are pregnant to exercise the same caution as a woman who knows she is pregnant. Women who are sexually

Drug Use During Pregnancy[3]

Drug Name	Effect on Fetus	Safe Use of Drug
NICOTINE	Heavy smoking can lead to low-birth-weight babies, which means that the baby may have more health problems. Especially harmful during second half of pregnancy.	Should be avoided.
ALCOHOL	Daily drinking of more than 2 glasses of wine or a mixed drink can cause "fetal alcohol syndrome": babies tend to low birth weight, mental retardation, physical deformity, and behavioral problems including hyperactivity, restlessness, and poor attention spans.	Should be avoided.
ASPIRIN	During last 3 months of pregnancy frequent use may cause excessive bleeding at delivery, and may prolong pregnancy and labor.	Under doctor's supervision.

Drug Name	Effect on Fetus	Safe Use of Drug
TRANQUILIZERS	Taken during the first 3 months of pregnancy, may cause cleft lip or palate or other congenital malformations.	Avoid if you might become pregnant and during early pregnancy. Use only under doctor's supervision.
BARBITURATES	Mothers who have taken large doses may have babies who are addicted. Babies may have tremors, restlessness, and irritability.	Only under doctor's supervision.
AMPHETAMINES	May cause birth defects.	Only under doctor's supervision.
MARIJUANA	Unknown.	Should be avoided.

active and may conceive are also wise to be very selective about the drugs they take. A woman who is trying to conceive should exercise the same degree of caution as a woman who is already pregnant. These women should inform any doctor that may prescribe medication that they are trying to conceive and might become pregnant at any time. Don't forget the dentist.

Pregnant women should keep careful records of all drugs taken during that time and make sure to include any OTCs. Remember the thalidomide and DES nightmares in which serious birth defects were caused by these drugs. The effects were not known until years later and officials are still trying to contact some of the mothers who took these drugs. The FDA has noted that "No drugs have been proven 100% safe for the unborn and we can't say there is no risk. Some risks are so small we can't detect them in laboratory or clinical trials." As a result aspirin and hundreds of thousands of other OTCs will have to carry the following warning as of December 3, 1983: "As with any drug, if you are pregnant or nursing a baby, seek the advice of a health professional before using this product." As many as 300,000 products may be affected by this new standard warning. Up until this decision by the FDA, only a limited number of nonprescription drugs had carried warnings to pregnant or nursing women.

Storage and dating. It is vitally important to know how to store medications (prescription and OTC). The first thing to keep in mind is that almost any drug, particularly adult-strength drugs, can act as a poison if taken by a curious young child. Childproof container caps can sometimes be a royal pain, but you should have no doubt about their being responsible for saving young lives. So use them, and do not keep medicine bottles or vials laying around unopened. Although a skull and crossbones is a universally accepted signal of danger among adults, it may serve more as an object of fascination to a young child. Your local poison control center can give you a sticker which in my part of the country is commonly referred to as "Mr. Yuk." The label is green in color and looks like this:

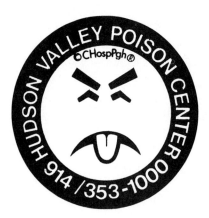

Young children seem to get the message that the stuff inside any container with a picture of Mr. Yuk on it must really taste horrible (yucky) and are less likely to put it in their mouths. You can put Mr. Yuk stickers on cleaning fluids and other poisons as well. Accidental poisoning is the fifth most common cause of death in the United States, with about 80 percent of all poisonings hitting children. Child poisoning is the most common pediatric emergency after trauma. Dr. Daniel Spyker of the University of Virginia's Blue Ridge Poison Center warns that you should not automatically follow antidote instructions on labels. The New York City Poison Control Project examined the labels of more than 1,000 common household products including cleansers, polishes, laundry products, drain openers, OTCs, insecticides, and car-care products. More than 85 percent of the instructions examined proved inadequate, incorrect, or dangerous. While new studies show that water may speed absorption of some poisons, milk will dilute any toxic substance without causing further damage. Keep a supply of ipecac, a syrup that induces vomiting, but it's best not to induce vomiting without the advice of a poison center. Be sure to have the phone number for your local poison control center, emergency squad, police, and hospital where you can read them in a hurry. You don't want to have to start looking up phone numbers in a real emergency. A good place to keep these numbers is pasted right on your phone or next to it. Possible poisoning, by the way, is another very important reason for knowing the names (generic and brand) and dosage strength of all the medications in your home. Those of you who live in rural and suburban areas should become familiar with poisonous plants. Contact your local poison control center for a list (with diagrams) of such plants.

Don't keep any medications in the bathroom medicine cabinet. The heat and humidity from showers, baths, and sink water cause drugs to deteriorate and spoil faster. The heat and humidity can even get inside those childproof containers. They tend to be airtight but not airproof, and spoilage does occur. Most drugs will do fine in a cool, dry place. Be sure to ask your doctor and/or pharmacist for storage instructions for every medication (including OTCs).

Some drugs remain chemically "pure" and effective over considerable periods of time. Others may deteriorate and spoil a lot sooner. It is important to know the "shelf life" of all medications. Some products are dated and read "Do not use after ———[date]." Others do not have such label instructions. Ask your doctor and/or pharmacist for this information. Throw out all drugs that have expired (flush them down the toilet). When in doubt, it is safer to discard the medication than to hold on to it. Look in your medicine cabinet. If you have drugs that are out-of-date, or have no label (so you are not sure what they are), or you really never use—throw them away. Most of us tend to hold on to every drug we ever bought. It doesn't make sense to hoard drugs that may be ineffective. Ask your doctor for some guidance as to what constitutes a sound family medicine cabinet. The odds are that you are overstocked with unnecessary and outdated drugs. No matter where you store your medications, *keep them out of the reach and view of young children!*

Contraindications. There are existing conditions or diseases that will not permit the use of certain drugs. The term used to warn the doctor, pharmacist, and consumer is *contra* (against) *indication* (to point out). Another way of stating this is: any symptom or circumstance indicating the inappropriateness of a form of treatment which is otherwise advisable. Some contraindications are stern in their warnings and are called "absolute." These absolute warnings are given to prevent the use of a drug that would expose the patient to extreme hazard. Other contraindications are milder and are called "relative." A relative warning does not completely forbid the use of the drug but certainly requires that special consideration be given to the decision to use it. This is a good example of how the benefits and risks need to be weighed together. Let's use oral contraceptives as an example of the two types of contraindications. There are more than twenty-five brand-name oral contraceptives sold in the United States. A phrase that is commonly used to indicate an absolute contraindication is "This drug should not be taken if. . . ." In the case of the oral contraceptives, this drug should not be taken if

- you have ever had or are now experiencing any form of phlebitis, embolism, stroke, angina, or heart attack;

168

- you have either impaired liver function or active liver disease (common in alcoholism);
- you have ever had cancer of the breast or reproductive organs;
- you suffer from abnormal and unexplained vaginal bleeding;
- you are allergic to either of the drugs (estrogen and progestin) contained in the brand you wish to purchase (check the label).

The phrase associated with relative contraindications is "Inform your doctor before taking this drug if. . . ." In the case of the oral contraceptives, inform your doctor before taking this drug if

- you have ever had an unfavorable reaction of any kind to any oral contraceptive;
- you have high blood pressure;
- you have a history of asthma or heart disease;
- you have epilepsy;
- you have cystic disease of the breasts;
- you have fibroid tumors of the uterus;
- you have a history of migraine headaches;
- you have diabetes or a tendency to diabetes;
- you smoke more than fifteen cigarettes a day;
- you have a history of endometriosis;
- you plan to have surgery within one month or less.

As you can see, contraindications are an important part of the decision-making process regarding whether or not to use a specific drug or entire drug family. (In fairness to the pill, it now appears that it may protect many women against two forms of cancer and other ailments.)

Food and drink while taking drugs. Just as some drugs don't mix well together, certain foods and drinks don't mix well either when you are undergoing drug therapy. Let's start with the simple stuff.

When you are given a prescription (or an OTC product is recommended by your physician or pharmacist), ask what liquid should be used to swallow that pill or wash down that elixir. Plain water is usually okay, but it's a good idea to know if other liquids (juice, soda or pop, milk) can be used safely. Some drugs should be washed down with a lot of water (like antibiotics, as a rule), while others require just a sip or two. The next thing you will want to know is whether the drug should be taken before, during, or after a meal. If it's before or after, find out how long before or how long after. Food helps some drugs to be absorbed into the body, while it does not help others. Doctor doesn't seem to know? Then ask him or her to find out, or ask your pharmacist. Don't leave it to chance!

The next thing you need to know is whether or not there are any restrictions to your diet during the drug therapy. For example, when the more commonly used tricyclic antidepressants don't work, doctors (psychiatrists in particular) will often make use of the MAO (monoamine oxidase) inhibitors. Included among the MAO inhibitors are Nardil (phenelzine), Marplan (isocarboxazid), and Parnate (tranylcypromine). All of these drugs must be combined with a carefully restricted diet. The reason is that the MAO inhibitors must not be allowed to combine with a substance called tyramine. The combination causes a severe elevation in blood pressure which can lead to very strong hypertensive headaches and stroke. Some of the foods and drinks containing tyramine are chicken liver, pickled herring, cheddar cheese, coffee, figs, chocolate, yogurt, beer, sherry, and Chianti wine.

Combining alcohol with many medications can lead to real trouble. The most serious trouble comes from mixing alcohol (a liquid sedative) with solid-state sedative drugs like the barbiturates (Seconal, Tuinal, phenobarbital), hypnotics (Dalmane, Quāālude), and tranquilizers (Miltown, Librium, Valium). These drug combinations quickly lead to overdosing. The main danger is that their effects are additive and can lead to depression (oversedation) of the central nervous system, causing anything from drowsiness to death. Antihistamines (Actifed, Allerest, Benadryl, Dristan, Dimetapp, to name a few) can make you feel drowsy and sedated. If you add alcohol to this, you are increasing the sedative effect. So whether your antihistamine comes in prescribed or OTC form, don't mix it with alcohol if you plan to drive or operate machinery.

Limited activities. Ever catch yourself saying something like this: "I'm too busy to be sick" or "I'll just work my way through this allergy season"? Many people just can't be bothered with being ill or suffering from conditions which tend to slow them down. That's one of the main reasons people use drugs as medicine. Over $500 million are spent by Americans each year on over-the-counter drugs alone to try to counteract the effects and symptoms of the common cold. Each year $5 billion are lost in wages and productivity due to the cold. Most OTC cold remedies (and there are many) contain antihistamines in varying amounts and types. Antihistamines like Benadryl (diphenhydramine hydrochloride) are also hypnotics, or sleep inducers, and allergy sufferers are warned not to drive, operate machinery, or fly a plane while taking this drug. However, since the common cold is caused by a virus (or combination of viruses) and is not an allergy, the cold remedies containing antihistamines are useless.

Some drugs have side effects which can lead to a change in activities. For example, the MAO inhibitors used to treat depression, such as Nardil, Marplan, and Parnate, while they may help with many of the major depressive symptoms, also can put a real damper on your sex life. Some of the sexual dysfunctions associated with these drugs are impotence, problems with urination, impaired ejaculation (men), and delayed orgasm (women). Some sexual dysfunction can occur with the tricyclic antidepression medications as well. Some drugs do not permit people to have much exposure to the sun (such as the phenothiazines used to treat psychosis).

Be sure to ask your doctor if there will be limitations to your usual activity regimen when drugs are being prescribed. If your activities have to be limited, take this as part of your course of treatment. If you are ill you cannot expect to operate at 100 percent of capacity. Admit you are human and take it easy.

Drug interactions. The body is always striving toward an ideal state which doctors call homeostasis (a state of equilibrium of the body's internal environment). A wide variety of biochemicals naturally exist in the human body and work toward that ideal. In recent years scientists have discovered naturally produced opiatelike substances in the central nervous system called endorphins. It is the endorphins that probably bring about a state called the "runner's high." While helping to counteract the pain of distance running, the endorphins produce an interesting "side effect": they cause the runner to feel "high" and exhilarated.

When things go wrong with our bodies (illness or some condition), science seeks to provide what nature often cannot. What is important to understand here is that once you start taking medicine (prescription or OTC) you are already causing a drug interaction. The interaction occurs between naturally existing body chemicals and the drugs you have introduced into your body in the form of medicine. If you take one medical drug (with its multiple actions), the body will accommodate and combine with this drug. The desired effect is relief from suffering. Side effects may have to be tolerated. We hope no adverse reactions occur. Therefore, as a general rule of thumb, the fewer drugs we take the better. The fewer drugs we take simultaneously, the better. This greatly reduces the chance for adverse reactions.

We have already considered food/drug interactions and drink/drug interactions. Now you must consider drug/drug interactions. When you mix drugs together, one and one don't always equal two. In some cases the effects are directly additive, as with booze and barbiturates (both sedatives). In other cases the drug combination produces an effect which neither alone could produce, or an effect may result which is greater than the total effects of each agent acting by itself. If you were to combine diazepam (Valium) with alcohol (two or more drinks), you could get so stoned that it would feel as if you had taken 50 milligrams of the drug instead of only 5, because of the additive sedative effect. In the extreme it can result in coma and death. There are other interactions which can be harmful. If you mix Flagyl (metronidazole), an antimicrobial drug used to treat infections like vaginitis, with alcohol you can expect nausea, stomach cramps, vomiting, and headaches. If you combine aspirin with an anticoagulant like Coumadin (warfarin), you could die from severe hemorrhaging. There are many other interactions, too numerous to mention here.

Keep in mind that nicotine can cause some drugs to break down chemically in the body more quickly. According to the 1979 Surgeon General's Report on Smoking and Health, ". . . Smoking of tobacco should be considered one of the primary sources of drug interaction in man."

Smoking and coffee drinking seem to go together. In one study, it was found that smokers metabolize the caffeine in coffee twice as fast (three hours as opposed to six) as nonsmokers. As smoking can influence the metabolism of many other drugs as well, make sure you inform the doctor that you are a smoker.

How to Avoid Negative Drug-to-Drug Interactions

1. When your doctor prescribes medicine, ask him or her if there are any specific other drugs to avoid. Ask about party drugs, tobacco, alcohol, and OTCs as well.

2. If it becomes necessary to take another medication, call your doctor to make sure that the two can be combined safely.

3. Keep in mind that another good reason to tell your doctor about drugs you are already taking is that they can significantly alter the results of laboratory tests. You don't need drugs masking a problem that is really there or creating the apparent existence of a condition that is not really there.

4. Don't take anyone else's medications on top of your own.

5. Try to keep the number of drugs you take to as few as possible.

6. Create a home reference library of relevant books (see the annotated bibliography for suggestions).

Practicing medicine without a license. The person sitting next to you at work acts just the way you do when you are uptight and nervous. So you offer him one of your Valium tablets. *Wrong!* You are at a party and develop a splitting headache. Your hostess, wishing to relieve your pain, offers you one of her Fiorinal with codeine (main ingredient, butalbital). You have taken Fiorinal *without* codeine (main ingredient, phenacetin) before for a headache, so you figure "Why not?" and you take it. *Wrong!* You could be in for a real surprise when the codeine mixes with the alcohol you consumed just a little while before—codeine increases the effects of sedatives like alcohol.

Only your doctor, together with you, can weigh all the relevant factors to be considered when taking drugs as medicine. Don't give your medicine to anyone else and don't take medicine prescribed for anyone else—the results could be disastrous. Leave the prescribing to the professionals. Your friends may give you drugs you don't need or that can harm you. You should not press your physician to give you drugs you do not need.

Stopping medications. If you want to stop smoking cigarettes on your own, you will be in good company, as 95 percent of those who quit did so on their own. But knowing when and how to stop taking prescription (and even some OTC) medications is something for which you need your doctor's advice. For example, Barbara Gordon describes in her book *I'm Dancing as Fast as I Can* what can happen when a person suddenly stops taking Valium after using it daily for years. The physical and psychological withdrawal effects can be really nasty and dangerous. Many drugs, like Valium, require step-down, or gradually decreasing, doses to ease any possible withdrawal effects. Allow your doctor to establish a detoxification protocol for any drug you are planning on stopping. If your doctor seems uncertain, tactfully ask him or her to get the information from a reliable source.

Do not stop taking a drug on whim—check it out with your doctor first. If you fail to fill a prescription for some reason, tell your doctor.

Stocking the medicine cabinet. Overstocking medicine cabi-
nets should be avoided. Your medicine chest should include only
those health-care products likely to be used on a regular basis.
The *FDA Consumer* and *Consumers' Research Magazine* recommend the following suggested items that will meet the needs of
most families:

Nondrug Products

- adhesive bandages of assorted sizes
- sterile gauze in pads and a roll
- absorbent cotton
- adhesive tape
- elastic bandage
- small blunt-end scissors
- tweezers
- fever thermometer
- hot water bottle
- heating pad
- eye cup for flushing objects out of the eye
- ice bag
- dosage spoon (common household teaspoons are rarely
  the correct dosage size)
- vaporizer or humidifier
- first aid manual

Drug Items

- analgesic-aspirin and/or acetaminophen. Both reduce fever and relieve pain, but only aspirin can reduce inflammation.
- emetic syrup of ipecac to induce vomiting. Read the instructions on how to use these products.
- antacid

- antiseptic solution
- hydrocortisone creams for skin problems
- calamine for poison ivy and other skin irritations
- petroleum jelly as a lubricant
- antidiarrhetic
- cough syrup—nonsuppressant type
- decongestant
- burn ointment
- antibacterial topical ointment

They further recommend antinausea medication if any family member is prone to motion sickness, a laxative, and some liniment. Seasonal items, such as insect repellents and sunscreens, round out the list.

Drugs and your children. While most illnesses in childhood are far from life-threatening and can be easily diagnosed and treated, most parents feel helpless when childhood illness occurs. One of the best ways to alleviate this parental anxiety is to become educated about responsible care for the sick child. As far as medication goes, the first guiding principle is that parents must assume responsibility for the use of all medicines that their children take! You will find helpful consultants in your doctors (pediatrician, internist, pediatric specialists) and your pharmacist, but as parent you take the direct role:

- to act as the facilitator of information between the child and the doctor.
- to teach your child the correct ways to use medicine.
- to make sure the medicine is taken properly and on time.
- to carefully monitor therapeutic progress and/or side effects.
- to prevent adverse reactions due to under- and overdosing (and other causes).
- to protect your child from ineffective and even dangerous medications (including OTCs). There are special dangers

176

to guard against for drugs that may impair normal development.

- to make sure that your children take their medicine, following the doctor's orders, even when extremely reluctant or when they are feeling better.
- to report any side effects, adverse reactions, overdoses and paradoxical effects to the doctor immediately. Paradoxical effects occur when a drug acts in a manner opposite to the one intended, such as a sedative acting as a stimulant.
- to ensure that contraindications are observed (there are many for children under twelve years of age).

There are drugs that represent a clear and present danger to children, and yet they are still on the market and some doctors are still prescribing them. Tetracycline belongs to the antibiotic family of drugs. Even though warnings have been accompanying all tetracycline preparations since 1972, some doctors are still prescribing them for children. Here is what the warning says:

The use of drugs of the tetracycline class during tooth development (last half of pregnancy, infancy, and childhood to the age of 8 years) may cause permanent discoloration of the teeth (yellow-gray-brown). This adverse reaction is more common during long-term use of the drugs but has been observed following repeated short-term courses. Enamel hypoplasia (malformation of teeth) has also been reported. Tetracyclines, therefore, should not be used in this age group unless other drugs are not likely to be effective or are contraindicated.

This class of drugs also has a long list of mild and serious adverse reactions. Side effects may include infections, often due to yeast organisms which can occur in the mouth, intestinal tract, rectum, and/or vagina, resulting in rectal and vaginal itching. Clearly for children under nine years of age, the risks far outweigh the benefits.

Brand-Name Antibiotics Containing Tetracycline

Achromycin	Sumycin
Mysteclin-F	Tetracycline HCL
Panmycin	Tetracycline syrup
Robitet	Tetracyn
SK-Tetracycline syrup	Tetrastatin
and capsules	Topicycline

This is just one example of drugs which are clearly contraindicated for younger children. Children also should not take cold remedies containing alcohol or antihistamines without specific directions from your doctor. It is a good idea for children to avoid combination-ingredient OTCs in general: (1) the doses may be wrong for children, (2) the ingredients may be ineffective, (3) the ingredients may mask symptoms which can warn you of a more serious health problem, and (4) the more ingredients, the greater the chances of side effects and adverse reactions. At least check with your pharmacist before purchasing OTCs for your child. If he or she is not sure about its safety or effectiveness for a child, *don't buy it!*

Remember, most illnesses run their course and disappear without any help from medication. More often than not it is your desire to provide instant relief to the suffering child that leads to the taking of too many or unnecessary drugs. Many pediatricians have "phone hours" which can save you the cost of an office visit.

When the dosage instructions tell you to administer a "teaspoon" of medicine, be careful! The common household teaspoon can vary in size from 2.5 to 9 milliliters. The recommended medical teaspoon is 5 milliliters. Ask your pharmacist to provide you with one of these accurate measuring instruments to ensure accuracy of dosage. It's a good idea to shake the bottle when the medication comes in liquid form to ensure mixing of all the ingredients. When pouring medications into measuring cups, do it at eye level and put a fingernail on the level you wish to fill to—both aid in accuracy.

Children vary greatly in size and weight. Two children may be the same age but one can be small and thin while the other is tall and heavy. The most accurate dosages are those that are computed by body-weight equivalents. Ask your doctor how your child's physique affects medication dosages.

Keep a written record of all side effects and adverse reactions that your child has to any drug, both prescription and OTC. Report these to your doctor as well. When it is time for a new medication, you can help by reminding your doctor of any of these negative effects.

Drugs taken by infants and young children must be monitored carefully for any possible impairment of normal growth and development. As mentioned previously, you should find out what food and drink is to be avoided while your child is undergoing drug therapy.

Let's take a look at the human side of administering medicine to your child.

1. Be matter-of-fact. Don't make a big deal out of it. There is no reason to apologize. Act as though you expect your child to be both courageous and cooperative.

2. Be honest. Don't tell them it tastes good when it really does not. Tell them it is medicine (even if it tastes like candy). Kids often ask if "it tastes bad." It helps if you know how it actually tastes. One response can be "It tastes like black cherry to me; how do you think it tastes?"

3. If physical restraint becomes necessary, don't display angry feelings, and get it over with as quickly as possible.

4. When mixing medicines in a drink, it's a good idea not to use things which your child drinks often. They may then resist that item in the future, even when it doesn't contain medicine.

5. Kids have a right to explanations that are geared to their age and comprehension. Keep it simple.

6. Tears are part of illness and sometimes of taking medicine. A little reassurance and love can go a long way. Guilt does not help a parent who is doing exactly what should be done to alleviate the illness.

7. If you react negatively to the medicines that you as an adult have to take, don't be surprised if your kids have the same reaction to their medicine.

8. If you combine the medicine with some food (like applesauce), don't give the child too much food. Illness usually causes a diminished appetite (and you want them to swallow all the medicine).

9. If you can crush the pill or capsule and mix it with food, this will help. It takes time to learn how to swallow a whole pill.

10. If the child gives you a hard time, lengthy negotiations are not a good idea. The medicine is for the child's health and well-being and therefore is not negotiable. If it becomes a real ordeal, consult your pediatrician for advice.

Sometimes our children are introduced in very innocent ways to the "high" that drugs can produce. One evening as we were seated around the dinner table, my son began describing his experiences with "space breath." When we all reacted with "What is space breath?" he reminded us of how, when seven years old, he was introduced to a new dentist who made a game of "astronauts" out of his initial visit. The office became a space ship, the chair became a couch in the rocket, and the mask which dispensed the nitrous oxide (laughing gas) became (in my son's imagination) "space breath." My daughter reacted to this hilarious story by stating how much she enjoyed using the "sweet air," as the dentist calls it. Nitrous oxide is a general-acting inhalant anesthetic and works by helping the central nervous system block the perception of pain (while drilling or cleaning). It leads to an altered state of consciousness, not unlike marijuana, causing feelings of giddiness, lightheadedness, and mild hallucinations. Its effects wear off very quickly, and as used by dentists it is a safe drug. But if you don't want your kids to get stoned at the dentist's office, then you may want to ask him or her to skip the "space breath" and use Novocain instead.

Drugs and older people. Homeostatis is the body's attempt to operate at a "steady state," or a state in which everything is in balance. As we grow older it becomes more difficult for the body to operate in this steady state, and this renders some bodily tissues more susceptible and sensitive to the actions of many drugs. So during the earliest and later years of life we must exercise special cautions in the use of all drugs as medicines— both prescription and OTC. Some of the changes that the body goes through in aging that directly affect the way it handles drugs are: (1) problems in the digestive system which change the way in which drugs are absorbed by the body, (2) reduced functioning of the liver and kidneys which makes it harder for the body to eliminate and metabolize (chemically break down) many drugs, (3) changes in the responsiveness of the nervous and circulatory systems which may mean smaller drug doses are required, to avoid reaching toxic levels, and (4) impairments in mental functioning such as memory which make the proper taking of medicines more problematic.

Retired people make up about 11 percent of the population but receive 25 percent of dispensed prescriptions. Adverse reactions occur three times more frequently in our older population. More than 85 percent of elderly ambulatory patients and 95 percent of elderly institutionalized patients receive drugs, 25 percent of which may be ineffective or unneeded. More than 70 percent of one elderly population study used nonprescription drugs without the knowledge of their primary-care provider.

It is not easy for an older person to shake off side effects and adverse reactions, and the drug therapy can become downright debilitating to an otherwise vital individual. The weighing of risks and benefits must be most carefully considered along with the careful selection of a dosage schedule. Some older people living alone may require assistance in following drug treatment therapies. Also, it is very common to find older persons involved in the use of more than one drug at the same time. The problems associated with this are negative drug interactions, greater risk of side effects and adverse reactions, interference with laboratory tests (possibly masking or delaying accurate diagnosis), and increased cost to the patient (many of whom live on fixed incomes).

Guidelines for Older People Taking Medications

1. Make sure the drug therapy is really indicated. For example, older people need less sleep, and what appears to be insomnia may be quite normal in the developmental sequence of aging.

2. Taking several drugs at a time is not a good idea. Make sure that your regular doctor knows all the drugs you are taking (including caffeine, nicotine and alcohol).

3. Since older people's bodies can't tolerate the same dosage and strength as younger people's, it's a very good idea to establish tolerance by starting with smaller-than-standard doses. Some doctors may even provide a free sample to test for side effects before putting you through the expense of a filled prescription.

4. Use easy-off caps and lids. Avoid childproof containers, as arthritis can make opening a medicine container a painful ordeal or even impossible.

5. Don't take drugs in a dimly lit room. Read the label carefully, and make sure you are taking what you are supposed to and in the right amount.

6. If you have trouble with your vision, ask the pharmacist to type the labels in all capital letters. Make sure the drug name and instructions are readable.

7. Ask your doctor for simple dosage instructions. Whenever possible, a single daily dose is preferable. As you grow older dosages usually need to be changed. Ask your doctor about this. Take nothing for granted. Ask lots of questions.

8. Many medications can be prepared in liquid form. Avoid large pills (tablets and capsules) if simpler dosage forms are available.

9. Sometimes people forget what they have taken or when they took it. The only drugs that should be kept at a bedside are emergency drugs like nitroglycerine. To avoid these problems, read labels carefully and keep a daily written record of what you took and when you took it.

10. Know the expiration dates of your drugs. It is important to discard outdated drugs.

11. Do not be embarrassed to discuss costs with your doctor and pharmacist. Generic drugs can often be substituted for the more expensive brand names. Different drugstores charge different amounts for drugs (of all kinds), so a little comparison shopping is in order. Pick pharmacies where you can get questions answered as well.

One of the problems faced by older people is loneliness. Another is boredom. People seek to counteract these unpleasant realities through an altered state of consciousness, i.e., by getting stoned. Older people use alcohol and prescription medications as well as OTCs to alter their moods. Some even use recreational and street drugs when they can get them. This is a risky business at best, often leading to dangerous and deadly drug combinations. Drug abuse and habituation are not only problems of the young.

If you care about your older relatives and friends, then you can possibly do them a big favor by having a serious discussion with them about the drugs in their life. By following your own common sense and the guidelines listed here you may help someone to (1) avoid unnecessary and harmful or ineffective drugs, (2) find a doctor and pharmacist who are cooperative in answering patients' questions about their medications, (3) avoid abusing drugs, (4) keep drugs from ruining the quality of their lives, and (5) learn to accept the realities of growing older without seeking "magic" from pills.

THE PHARMACIST

So far our emphasis has been on responsible self-care coupled with a good working relationship with your doctor(s). A modern-day partnership around drugs as medicine must include a third, equally important, member: the pharmacist. When you make use of both consultants as advisers on drugs, you are taking advantage of the best of both worlds—medicine and pharmacology. Many of you will remember, sometimes with a good deal of affection and nostalgia, the friendly and helpful neighborhood druggist. He knew your whole family and everyone else in the neighborhood. People often approached him with intimate concerns about health, in some cases instead of the doctor. He was someone you trusted with your health and felt a certain closeness with. Contrast that with the modern pharmacy. Often it is part of a large chain; the store sells many things besides medications; the pharmacists are hidden behind a bullet-proof barrier or on a raised platform (both of which diminish any chance for private conversation); you don't know their names and they don't know yours; in short, the whole arrangement has changed for the worse. Hospital pharmacy, interestingly enough, has been moving in the opposite direction. Pharmacists have come out from behind their cages, participate in rounds with the doctors, meet with patients, and are a more involved part of the hospital treatment team. The more doctors in hospitals interact with pharmacists, the more they come to value their input into the patient's total care plan.

The pharmacist who owns or works in a profit-making drugstore has an inherent conflict. He is a trained professional with a good working knowledge of the latest in drug effectiveness and safety. But he has to choose between his profit motive and his ethical sense of what's good for the consumer. For example, he is often forced to choose between selling you a more expensive name-brand product and a less expensive but equally effective generic drug. Or he may have to choose between selling you an ineffective over-the-counter product and suggesting that you not purchase that item. He is also under a lot of pressure from drug manufacturers to purchase, stock, and prominently display their products. The manufacturer's representative is more interested in products that sell than in their therapeutic benefits. (Drug companies routinely sell products not approved in the United

States to other nations where less rigorous standards permit their sale. One manufacturer marketed to an African nation infant formula that American officials would not permit to be used by babies in this country!) Drug manufacturers provide only the minimum required information about side effects and adverse reactions on their packaging, while the pharmacist may know much more that the patient should be told. The pharmacist finds himself faced by many ethical dilemmas, but many have solved these in favor of the consumer without hurting their profits. Shop around for the ethical pharmacist. You should choose him or her with the same care as you do your doctor, in terms of both competence and morality.

Choosing a Pharmacist

1. You want someone you can talk to. The pharmacist should be patient and understanding. If he or she is too busy to talk with you, find someone who will.
2. Pharmacists should be a source of expert information concerning types of drugs, side effects, adverse reactions, contraindications, efficacy of products, etc. And they should be willing to share this information with you both verbally and in writing. They should be happy to answer your questions—no matter how silly or naive you think they sound.
3. Keep this ideal in mind when choosing a pharmacist: "Your pharmacist should provide you with safe and effective medications at the lowest rate of cost."
4. Good pharmacists don't stock really lousy products in their stores.
5. Good pharmacists will steer you away from a product they feel is not good for you, even if it means losing a sale.
6. One of the best ways that pharmacists can be of help to an individual patient is to keep a record or profile on each of their customers. The profile should include both prescription and OTC information.
7. A good pharmacist will attend to you personally, giving you information about how to take the medicine and side effects

to watch out for. Some pharmacies even provide this information in writing.

8. If the pharmacist has any questions about what the doctor has prescribed, he or she should not hesitate to contact the doctor.

9. An ethical business person tempers the need to make a living with a careful guarding of their professional reputation.

Drug prices vary considerably, not only between generic and brand-name drugs, but also between pharmacies. As drug prices are presently increasing at the rate of about 7 to 10 percent a year, this can become an important part of your budget. However, price alone does not make a good pharmacy. It is definitely worth a few extra dollars a year to find a pharmacist who really meets the criteria we've defined.

The best approach to drug therapy is a situation where:

1. The doctor is clear and explicit in advising the patient about the drug to be used—intended benefits, known side effects, dosage instructions, and so on.

2. The pharmacist assists and reinforces the directions given by the doctor and answers any questions the patient has.

3. The patient has used both consultants and clearly understands the intentions of the therapy and what to do if problems arise.

If any of the ingredients are missing, problems can occur. If you are a hospital patient and a regimen of drug therapy is being prescribed, ask lots of questions and don't hesitate to ask that a pharmacist be made available to speak with you if you so desire. For example, many patients in hospitals are routinely given orders for sleep medication before anyone (including the doctor) knows if they will have trouble sleeping. If you don't want or need a medication, discuss it with the doctor and the pharmacist. Some hospital pharmacies are now providing both in-patients and out-patients with "patient package inserts," which patients can read and thereby learn more about what they are taking and how to take it. This is particularly useful when patients leave the hospital. Some hospital pharmacies operate telephone services which give out drug information, and some operate poison hotlines. These are valuable services and you should have their phone numbers within easy reach in case of emergency. Your neighborhood pharmacist should be willing to answer phone inquiries as well. If he won't, find one who will.

THE "DATED" PHYSICIAN

"Drug mills" are operated by unscrupulous doctors who only want to make money at the expense of the practice of good medicine. "Doctor Feelgoods" supply their patients (for a handsome fee) with stimulants, sedatives, narcotics, tranquilizers, hypnotics, ad nauseam. My wife, a registered nurse, had occasion to act as a private-duty nurse for a wealthy couple in their late sixties whose rear ends were completely shot out by four decades of Demerol (a powerful synthetic narcotic) addiction. The drug and hypodermic needles had been faithfully supplied by their doctor during this entire time period. The two patients whined like street junkies when their medication was late in coming.

Psychiatrists appear to be overrepresented among impaired (chemically dependent) physicians for both alcoholism and drug addiction. State medical societies are working on legislation and guidelines to protect the physician and the patient when impairment occurs. Doctors, just like the rest of society, have come to see drugs as quick and easy solutions for our ills. We are all brainwashed into believing that there is a "pill for every ill." Doctors are continuously having drugs of every conceivable description pushed at them by drug manufacturers' sales representatives. It's no wonder they succumb to the same drug maladies as the rest of us. If you have reason to suspect that your doctor is either impaired or indiscriminately pushing drugs, it's time to seek out a new doctor.

It is far easier to avoid drug mills and impaired physicians than it is to avoid a far more common phenomenon—the dated physician. It is important to understand that many different subjects must be covered in medical school curricula and that different disciplines and departments compete actively to get a piece of the action. Most medical students and physicians-in-training are exposed to a minimum of material on pharmacology—the study of drugs, their origin, nature, properties, and their effects on living organisms. They may be exposed to clinical pharmacology, which is the actual use of drugs on live patients, during their internship and residency. But few doctors learn much during the four years of medical school about the basic science of pharmacology which will enable them to keep apace of the information explosion in the field. The pharmacology they do study is sandwiched between so many other courses that it is certainly fair to assume that this subject matter does not receive a high priority in medical training. This is a shame, because the prescription of various medicines is most doctors' stock-in-trade.

How then do doctors keep up with the new drugs that are constantly coming into the marketplace? One way is through a publication called the *Physicians' Desk Reference (PDR)*. This large volume is the doctor's main source of information regarding drugs, including side effects, main actions, adverse reactions, contraindications, cautions, and the like. How do the various drugs get listed in this tome? The manufacturers pay to have their products listed in the *PDR*. The *PDR* is actually one large advertising venture. How else do doctors learn about drugs? They read the pharmaceutical companies' advertisements in a wide variety of medical journals. And finally, the major source of information for the practicing physician is the sales force of the drug manufacturers, called "detail people."

The main thrust of the *PDR,* the journal ads, and the detail persons is to sell drugs to the doctor. The detail people know how busy most doctors are and are only too happy to provide them with promotional materials lauding the purported benefits of their products (not to mention the free samples). Doctors prove to be just as gullible as the layman when it comes to some of the seductive claims and slick advertising coming at them from the drug companies. Dr. Richard Burack, author of *The New Handbook of Prescription Drugs,* comments:

> It is time to remind medical students, doctors-in-training, and all of the concerned public that the aims of the drug manufacturers are different from the aims of good doctors. The manufacturers wish to maximize their profits by encouraging doctors to write as many prescriptions as possible for the most expensive drugs. Manifestly, good doctors should minimize writing prescriptions and, as purchasing agents for patients, should do all they can to keep the cost of necessary medications as low as possible.[4]

A related problem is that doctors may fail to consider that nonmedicinal remedies may work as well as or better than those employing medicine. In 1979, an article in the *Journal of the American Medical Association* stated that:

> Although a complete picture of prescribing practices is not at hand, the conclusions of two influential groups of physicians and researchers who have studied the matter are that the average physician is insufficiently educated in clinical pharmacology, often misled by industry advertising and "detail men," and inadequately informed of the alternatives to pharmacological therapy.[5]

The discovery of a number of drugs and drug families has been of great value to the practice of modern biomedicine and surgery. But the simple truth is that there are very few breakthroughs. An awful lot of the so-called new drugs are in fact "me-too" products. When a drug company does discover a new drug, that drug may be patented, and the patent is good for seventeen years before its generic equivalent can be marketed and sold. Many of the me-too drugs have the exact same generic chemical ingredients in the same dosages but with different filler substances (used to bind the product). However, each company markets this drug under its own unique brand name and prices vary considerably. Where do doctors learn about these me-too drugs? From the same *Physicians' Desk Reference,* professional-journal ads, and detail people as all the other prescription drugs.

Do drug manufacturers always tell the truth in their advertisements? Consider the following examples regarding commonly used OTC products in the analgesic (pain-killing) family of drugs. The analgesic market represents approximately $1 billion per year.

Claim: Bufferin (manufactured by Bristol-Myers Co.) is "twice as fast as aspirin."

Fact: The only pain reliever in Bufferin is aspirin. Despite the fact that Bristol-Myers claims that Bufferin enters the bloodstream faster than plain or unbuffered aspirin, the company couldn't furnish the Federal Trade Commission with any significant medical evidence that the speed of aspirin absorption has anything to do with the speed of pain relief.

Claim: "New, improved" Bayer (manufactured by Sterling Drug Co.) is "better-tolerated than regular aspirin" and "There's never been an aspirin like it. Ever."

Fact: Bayer is nothing but regular aspirin. The coating on the product may make it easier to swallow, but that's all.

The FTC recently issued a cease-and-desist order against the American Home Products Corporation and its advertisement for Anacin and Arthritis Pain Formula. The order was upheld, upon appeal, by the federal courts. Michael Pertschuk, a member of the FTC, said, "I'm not going to say they're liars, but I am sure going to say they engaged in deception and created false impressions." Anacin ads have used phrasing like:

Claim: "Two Anacin tablets have more of the one pain reliever doctors recommend most than four of the other leading extra-strength tablets."

Claim: "Anacin starts with as much pain reliever as the leading aspirin tablet, then adds an extra core of this specific fast-acting ingredient against pain."

Claim: "Doctors know Anacin contains more of the specific medication they recommend for pain than the leading aspirin, buffered aspirin, or extra-strength tablet."

Fact: The extra level of pain reliever is more aspirin. According to FTC testimony, extra aspirin has no proven effect on the speed or quality of pain relief. The only thing that separates Anacin from store-brand aspirin is a pinch of caffeine, which has no pain-relieving qualities.

Why are the aspirin manufacturers so reluctant to disclose that the product they are selling is aspirin? According to Samuel Murphy, Jr., the lawyer who argued American Home Products' case before the court: "I don't think it's a question of being reluctant to disclose. Most people know what's in the product. What you're trying to do in advertising is to get people's attention in a very short span of time." The FTC notes that aspirin "is so commonplace that a maker of one aspirin-based pain reliever seeking to differentiate its product from the rest faces a formidable marketing task. What better way to meet this challenge than to establish a new identity for the product dissociated from ordinary aspirin, and then to represent it as special and more effective than its competitors?" Caveat emptor—let the buyer beware!

Ours is a drug-taking society. The drug-seeking behavior is so ingrained in us that we are disappointed if we leave the doctor's office without at least one prescription for medicine to "cure" us. The physician's prescription writing is often a knee-jerk response, but so is our eagerness to be the recipients of the drugs (even to the extent that people can experience effects not caused by the pharmacologic agent—this is called the placebo effect). There are many cogs in the wheel that produces the dated physician. They are: (1) minimal training in basic and clinical pharmacology, (2) pressure from pushy and persuasive detail people,

(3) proliferation of me-too drugs and combination drugs, (4) pressure from pill-hungry patients, (5) lax enforcement of standards and guidelines by the Food and Drug Administration, (6) equally lax enforcement by the Federal Trade Commission regarding outrageous advertising claims, and (7) the information explosion in the pharmaceutical field. So we end up with a doctor with a threadbare start in pharmacology relying on profit-oriented sales people to provide you, the overanxious public, with a seemingly endless variety of medicines, only some of which are helpful.

Consumers and doctors alike look to federal regulatory agencies like the FDA to protect us from drugs that fall below established standards of effectiveness and safety. Yet one out of every eight prescriptions filled in the United States—169 million prescriptions, costing over $1.1 billion, in 1979—is for a drug not considered effective by the government's own standards. This lack of effectiveness means you are exposing yourself to risks that carry no benefits! In their revealing book *Pills That Don't Work*, Dr. Sidney Wolfe, Christopher M. Coley, and the Health Research Group (founded by Ralph Nader) report on 607 drugs considered ineffective by the FDA that, as of August 1980, were still on the market and still being prescribed by doctors. About two-thirds of these products are combinations, which means that while the risk of side effects increases proportionately, the benefits of these ineffective drugs does not increase at all. The reasons for their continued use: "Governmental inefficiency, lethargy and timidity, orchestrated by heavy pressure from drug companies to keep these drugs on the market." Even after the National Academy of Sciences National Research Council had ruled on the effectiveness of all prescription drugs approved for marketing between 1938 and 1962 (the year the drug laws were amended), it took a lawsuit by the American Public Health Association and the National Council of Senior Citizens to get the FDA to expedite the removal of these less-than-effective drugs from the marketplace.

What is the answer to this dilemma, of which the dated physician is only the tip of the iceberg? Nothing less than a massive campaign of drug education. The campaign must be mounted by a consortium of doctors, pharmacologists, consumers, pharmacists, and researchers. None of these people should be on the payroll of drug manufacturers! It is a requirement of most doctors that they participate in continuing educational programs in order to ensure continuing licensure. Drug updates must be part of a nationwide mandated curriculum for physicians. If the FDA were not so subject to budget cutting and political pressuring, perhaps it could meet its own mandate and help give us the protection we need. FDA guidelines on patient package inserts (PPIs) are now undergoing the same kind of foot-dragging that has characterized the removal of ineffective drugs. Some people are more interested in their own profits than in other people's health.

In January 1982 ABC News covered OTC cold remedies on their program *20/20*. Every year Americans spend millions of dollars seeking relief from cold symptoms. According to the experts interviewed by correspondent John Stossel, the only things that can help your cold are: (1) aspirin or a Tylenol-type substitute for pain, (2) a spray for your nose (watch out for "rebound"— the need to keep using them, leading to a functional addiction), and (3) dextromethorphan for a dry cough. Nothing else seems to work on a cold. This means that the manufacturers' claims for their products (particularly combination products) are all bunk! The claims are either exaggerated, patently false, suggest unneeded ingredients, or are otherwise misleading. Until the day that this massive educational campaign for doctors and the public is launched, and until the FDA and the FTC get their acts together, here are some questions you can ask your doctor to avoid the problem:

1. Have you prescribed this medication before? for my illness or condition? with what results?
2. Has the manufacturer made any claims for this drug which in your experience are unwarranted?
3. What is the research evidence that this drug is effective?
4. What reference materials (besides the *PDR*) do you use to keep abreast of the latest drug developments?

MANAGING THE DRUGS IN YOUR LIFE

5. Would you mind if I consulted my pharmacist about this drug?
6. When was the last time you took an update course on drugs?
7. Do you subscribe to any drug publications not produced by drug manufacturers (newsletters, bulletins, etc.)?

Be assertive. Doctors don't like these kinds of questions, but you can help your doctor to realize that as an informed patient you want him or her to be an informed doctor.

Another reason for being assertive with doctors and pharmacists to secure needed drug information is the way the federal government has been dragging its feet about patient package inserts (PPIs). Under the Carter administration the FDA had announced plans to require PPIs for 375 prescription drugs. Met with a furious uproar from the American Medical Association and the drug industry, the FDA reduced their plans to a pilot program involving only ten drugs. The Reagan administration suspended the pilot program in January 1981 and formally buried it in September 1982. In October 1982, with great fanfare the AMA in cooperation with a group called the United States Pharmacopeial Convention began a voluntary drive to provide instruction sheets written in plain language on twenty widely used medicines including tranquilizers, insulin, oral penicillin, and nitroglycerin. The program is costing $2.7 million, $1.8 million being donated by drug companies and the rest by the 240,000-member AMA. The Carter plan had been scuttled because the AMA claimed the language in some leaflets might frighten some patients into not taking the medicine. The new sheets are being touted as "honest, accurate, reflective of fact and yet not frightening."

WOMEN BEWARE!

I am a female alcoholic and I've been getting over on doctors for years. I've been diagnosed as schizophrenic, severely depressed, and a hysterical personality. I have suffered from neuritis, ulcers, gastritis, and a fatty liver. Over the years I have been given prescriptions for Thorazine, Compazine, Mellaril, Valium, Librium and God knows how many drugs for my physical problems. I have seen no less than eighteen doctors over a period of fifteen years and not a single one of them knew I was an alcoholic. Not one ever took an alcohol or drug history. Of course I wasn't going to volunteer my "drinking problem" to them, but damn it, they never asked, either! You know what these doctors did do for me? They got me cross-addicted!

When I first met Martha (not her real name) she was really strung out on booze and tranquilizers. After getting her detoxified from both drugs, I took her to an internist who knows about alcoholism and drug abuse, and I took her to her first meeting of Alcoholics Anonymous. I read her old medical records very carefully and could find plenty of evidence of alcoholism (hidden between the lines) and very little of major mental disorder that fit her behavior while dry and clean. Psychotherapy consisted of her making a long hard climb back to self-respect while going to A.A. almost daily for a year (she still is quite active). Her old doctors had mistaken a toxic psychosis caused directly by the alcohol and sedative pills for an actual schizophrenic break. Her depressions were understandable in terms of her heavy drinking and remorse over this drinking. Her hysteria was simply a cry of pain and a plea for help. Male physicians were too ready to see her as a weak and sick woman who just needed some medicine to make her all right. They gave her neither the time nor the respect she deserved and needed. What they did give her was prescriptions, sexist attitudes, and the short end of the medical stick. I wish Martha's story were the exception. I'm afraid it's much closer to being the rule. Looking at the way women are treated by various health-care professionals is a real eye-opener.

Item: A group of doctors in California wanted to know how male physicians would respond to five common medical complaints: back pain, headaches, dizziness, chest pain, and fatigue. What they found is that workups for these complaints were significantly more extensive for male than for female patients. The conclusion: male physicians tend to take illness more seriously in men than women.

Item: The House Select Committee on Narcotics Abuse and Control held hearings to discover why so many women were taking mood-altering drugs. They found that "thirty-two million (42%) women compared to 19 million (26%) men have used tranquilizers prescribed by a doctor. Sixteen million (21%) women as compared to 12 million (17%) men have used physician-prescribed sedatives and 12 million (17%) women as compared to 5 million (8%) men have used amphetamines ordered by a doctor. An estimated 9 million women use tranquilizers, 3 million women use sedatives, and 1 million women take their first stimulants prescribed by a doctor in any given year."

Item: A nationwide survey of more than 15,000 A.A. members showed that 29 percent of the women but only 15 percent of the men were addicted to other drugs besides alcohol. Of new A.A. members age thirty or younger, 55 percent of women were cross-addicted, compared to 36 percent of men.

Item: A landmark study in mental health asked a group of psychotherapists to define, respectively, a mature healthy man, a mature healthy woman, and a mature healthy adult. With a high degree of agreement the therapists defined a healthy mature woman as more submissive, less independent, less adventurous, less competitive, more excitable in minor crises, more easily hurt, and more emotional than a mature healthy man. A mature healthy adult was described in a manner remarkably similar to a man. The study results demonstrated a pervasive sexist attitude among therapists.

Item: In a study of staff and patient attitudes toward women in a drug-free therapeutic community treatment agency, staff viewed women as more emotional, more sensitive, limited by their biology, needing to please men, and implicitly "sicker" than men. Staff also placed greater emphasis on interpersonal relationships being uniquely female addict problems. A stable relationship with a man was thought by staff to be more important to success in treatment for a woman, while realistic job plans were considered more important to a man.

Item: In a study of attitudes toward women in a methadone maintenance program, the staff greatly underestimated the extent to which female clients felt unable to express their feelings, have bad feelings about their bodies, feel they are not smart, and feel they need more education. In brief, staff had more trouble perceiving the problems of their female clients than of their male clients. This was surprising considering the disproportionate number of women on the clinic staff.

Item: A number of separate studies have come to similar conclusions regarding drug advertising and women. Many of the drug ads suggest the use of mood-altering drugs as the best treatment for problems that are often beyond traditional medical and psychiatric concepts of illness. Many of the "problems" targeted in the drug ads are everyday life problems that could better be dealt with by psychotherapy, social action, or closer ties between people. Many ads portray women who supposedly can't cope with their "role" and women who "bother" their husbands and doctors. Rather than suggesting coping with or learning to handle these problems, the drug industry promotes the use of drugs to ease "anxiety."

Item: An examination of statistics on drug overdoses maintained by the National Institute on Drug Abuse shows that women continue to predominate over men. The highest percentage is found among white women and the lowest among white men. Most prominent among the drugs involved in emergency-room drug episodes are Valium, aspirin, Dalmane, Darvon, Elavil, and Librium.

Sexism has permeated the practice of medicine, pharmacotherapy, psychotherapy, and the treatment of drug and alcohol problems. Eighty-eight percent of all doctors are men. The number of women presently in medical school is increasing significantly (some 30 to 40 percent) but it will be some years before they join the ranks of practicing physicians.

Evaluating Mental-Health Programs and Therapists

Almost 90 percent of psychoactive medications are prescribed by doctors other than psychiatrists, mostly "general practitioners." The general practitioner relies on the prescription pad and has little training in mental health and quality-of-life issues, which leads to overprescribing, especially for women.

- Many doctors are "too busy" to give women patients the time needed to really hear the full context of the problems they are experiencing. Note the actual amount of time that you spend with the doctor on your next visit. Bet it doesn't take more than a few minutes for a cursory exam and a real quick chat, and you probably emerge with at least one prescription.
- Many doctors harbor a wide range of sexist attitudes, and because of this tend to see many problems in terms of women resisting the roles they ought to be content to fill. It goes something like this: "If you would just stay home and care for your husband and kids, everything would be fine. In the meantime here is a prescription for something to calm your nerves."
- Many doctors derive much of their perceived power from being able to provide instant relief through medication. It also keeps them from having to get involved in underlying issues. Thus, very often they tend to be ignorant of or otherwise ignore nondrug remedies to the problem.

A balance needs to be struck between the use of psychoactive medications and the use of other approaches and therapies that do not include drugs, such as psychotherapy, self-help, mutual support groups, anonymous societies such as Alcoholics Anonymous, and herbal, natural, and folk medicines.

Here are some general guidelines to help you in choosing practitioners and agencies that (a) may use drug therapy and (b) claim they can help you with an existing drug problem.

1. Problems exist in a context. Is the helper interested in hearing about your general situation? Willing to try to understand your problem within the context of your lifestyle? The problem may be personal, interpersonal, or impersonal in nature. Can the helper assist you in pinpointing sources of problems outside of yourself as well as within you?

2. What attitudes does he harbor about women in general? Does he believe that the rights and roles of women in society are to be restricted or expanded? Does he treat you as a person or a woman? Is he trying to force you into preconceived roles or is he helping you become what you want to be?

3. When considering drug therapy for psychological problems, is the drug therapy part of a total plan of treatment or the only service being offered? As a rule, drugs alone deal with symptoms. You will probably want to get to the underlying cause(s) and should therefore ask for more than a prescription for medication.

4. Is the helper willing to seriously consider nondrug alternatives? For example, many people have found that proper diet and exercise help with anxiety and stress in place of drugs. Does the helper respect your right not to take drugs?

Some specific considerations if drug therapy is being proposed:

1. Does your doctor give you adequate information about benefits and risks so that you feel you can make an informed decision?

2. Can the doctor suggest some relevant reading material on the drug before you make your decision? Can he

or she introduce you to anyone who has taken this drug and been helped?

3. How long will you have to take the drug? Will the doctor consider a "drug holiday" when the crisis is past to see how you manage on your own?

4. Is counseling or psychotherapy being recommended along with the medication, or is the drug being touted as a cure-all?

5. Is the doctor really familiar with your unique problem? Has he or she dealt with many cases like yours? Is the drug being recommended specific to your problem or is it a general "psychic panacea" for "nerves" and "uptight ladies"?

Choosing a drug treatment program:

1. Are there women on staff in clinical and administrative policy-making positions? Remember, everything falls from the top in organizations.

2. What is their track record in working with female clients? Can you talk with some of their women clients before enrolling?

3. If you wish, can your therapist or counselor be a woman?

4. Does your therapist respect your individual needs as opposed to treating you as just another woman with a drug problem?

5. If you want help with educational or vocational concerns, can they provide it? The ability to earn a living is a vital part of recovery for men and women.

6. Are they knowledgeable about your drug(s) of abuse? Some programs try to be all things to all people. Some do better with drug problems while others do better with alcoholism.

7. Is there an end point in treatment? Can you graduate into less intense treatment as you progress in your recovery?

8. Do they provide services for physical, psychological, and spiritual recovery? Do they understand the special needs of women and relate to them as an essential part of treatment?

Some problems do not need to be put into diagnostic categories and placed in the hands of professionals or paraprofessionals. Have you considered your own personal network of friends and associates? Many people are able to work things out or to get through a crisis by turning to a friend who will listen and care. Sisterhood can be very powerful indeed. You should explore self-help and support groups in your community like Alcoholics Anonymous (A.A.), Pills Anonymous (P.A.), consciousness-raising groups, Parents Anonymous (for child-abuse problems), Toughlove (for serious problems with adolescent children), programs sponsored by the National Organization for Women (NOW), and many others. The psychology committee of NOW's New York chapter has put together an informative guide entitled "A Consumer's Guide to Nonsexist Therapy," which deals with choosing a therapist and the rights of clients in therapy. You may also wish to contact local feminist organizations for listings of self-help and support groups in your area.

The task force on sex bias and sex role stereotyping in psychotherapeutic practice of the American Psychological Association has provided some excellent guidelines for therapy with women:

1. The conduct of therapy should be free of constrictions based on sex roles, and the options explored between you and the practitioner should be free of sex role stereotypes.
2. Your therapist should recognize the reality, variety, and implications of sex-discriminatory practices in society and should facilitate your examination of options in dealing with such practices.
3. Your therapist should be knowledgeable about current scientific findings on sex roles, sexism, and individual differences resulting from sex-defined identity.

4. The theoretical concepts employed by your therapist should be free of sex bias and sex role stereotypes.

5. Your therapist should demonstrate acceptance of women as equal to men by using language free of derogatory labels.

6. Your therapist should avoid establishing the source of personal problems within you when they are more properly attributable to situational or cultural factors.

7. Your therapist and you should mutually agree upon aspects of the therapy relationship such as treatment modality, time factors, and fee arrangements.

8. While the importance of the availability of accurate information to your family is recognized, the privilege of communication about diagnosis, prognosis, and progress ultimately resides with you, not with the therapist.

9. If authoritarian processes are employed as a technique, the therapy should not have the effect of maintaining or reinforcing stereotyped dependence of women.

10. Your assertive behaviors should be respected.

11. The therapist whose female clients are subjected to violence in the form of physical abuse or rape should recognize and acknowledge that the client is the victim of a crime.

12. Your therapist should recognize and encourage exploration of your sexuality and should recognize your right to define your own sexual preferences.

13. The therapist should not have sexual relations with a woman client nor treat her as a sex object.

When you are satisfied that you are in the hands of a competent nonsexist doctor who takes the time to understand your needs and situation, you should consider drug therapy as one of the resources available to you. Aside from the blatantly ineffective drugs, some medications can be a definite aid in some cases. Don't throw the baby out with the bath water. But make sure that you are an equal partner to the decision to enter into drug therapy with a full understanding of all the risks and benefits. Stand up for your rights as a woman and a consumer.

WARNING: THIS DRUG MAY BE HABIT FORMING!

Most people associate drug dependency and addiction with illegal street drugs. The legal status of a drug does not have a thing to do with its potential for becoming habit forming. Many prescription and OTC drugs have a potential for physical and psychological dependence. To understand addiction, we must start with some clearly defined terminology.

Tolerance: As your body adapts to drugs over time, certain tissues react less vigorously to the drug's presence. This cumulative resistance to the pharmacological effects of a drug is called tolerance. It occurs when the repeated use of a given dose produces a decreased effect. This means that the person will have to take increased doses to get the original effect.

Withdrawal: The cluster of characteristic reactions and behavior unique to the stopping (or severe reduction) of a specific drug. Different drugs create different withdrawal syndromes. Depending upon the drug, amount taken, and frequency of usage, withdrawal can range from mild to life-threatening. Physical addiction is required for withdrawal to occur.

Physical addiction: Physical addiction is evidenced by either tolerance or withdrawal symptoms. Since tolerance is actually brain tissue getting "used" to certain levels of a drug being present, withdrawal is the body's way of making a statement, which we commonly call craving. Withdrawal symptoms are caused by the body's trying to cope with a sudden upheaval in body chemistry.

Psychological addiction: This is the belief that one can't function properly or cope with the stresses of daily living without the drug in question. It is a compulsive need for a drug's mental effects; the user feels his or her well-being is threatened without it. Sometimes referred to as habituation, it may exist alone or with physical addiction.

Functional addiction: This is what is sometimes called a "medical" addiction. It happens when a drug effectively relieves an annoying or distressing condition and the body becomes increasingly dependent upon the action of that drug to maintain well-being. These drugs usually act on symptoms and do not involve the brain in creating altered states of mood or consciousness. Functional addiction is different from physical and psychological addiction.

According to the General Accounting Office, the investigative arm of Congress, the abuse of prescription drugs causes far more deaths than use of illegal drugs. "Millions of Americans abuse prescription drugs, often with tragic results," stated their report released in November of 1982. The federal Drug Abuse Warning Network showed that prescription drugs "dominate the statistics" on drug related deaths and emergencies. In 1980, prescription

Drug-Abuse Warning Network
Top 20 Controlled Drugs Abused
(Calendar Year 1980)

| | | | Drug mentions reported by | |
| | | | --- | --- |
Drug	Type	Controlled Substances Act Schedule	EMER- GENCY ROOMS Number	MEDICAL EXAM- INERS Number
Diazepam (Valium)	P	4	16,603	346
Heroin	I	1	8,487	885
Methaqualone	PT	2	5,958	137
Flurazepam (Dalmane)	P	4	4,538	92

Drug	Type	Controlled Substances Act Schedule	Drug mentions reported by	
			EMER-GENCY ROOMS Number	MEDICAL EXAM-INERS Number
Marijuana	I	1	4,513	10
PCP	I	2	4,441	43
Cocaine	I	2	4,153	265
D-Propoxyphene (Darvon)	P	4	2,964	326
Phenobarbital	P	4	2,861	225
Amphetamine	PT	2	2,658	37
Chlordiazepox-ide (Librium)	P	4	2,602	48
Methadone	P	2	2,500	376
Secobarbital/amobarbital	P	2	2,183	144
Acetaminophen w/codeine	P	3	1,980	5
Pentazocine (Talwin)	P	4	1,914	66
Ethchlorvynol (Placidyl)	P	4	1,834	103
Speed	PT	2	1,808	0
Chlorazepate (Tranxene)	P	4	1,719	5
Oxycodone (Percodan)	P	2	1,498	3
LSD	I	1	1,452	2
Total P & PT			53,620	1,913
Total I			23,046	1,205
Total			76,666	3,118

P—Prescription drug; normally found in the legitimate market
PT—Prescription-type drug; significant origins outside legitimate domestic market
I—Illegal drug
Drugs are listed by generic name (example, brand names are in parentheses)

drugs were identified in 3,535, or 74 percent, of 4,747 deaths attributed to drugs by medical examiners. In the same year hospital emergency room reports showed that 71,431, or 75 percent, of 95,502 drug emergencies were due to the misuse of prescription drugs. In that year, fifteen of the twenty drugs most frequently mentioned were prescription as opposed to illegal drugs. The table above shows the distribution of these drugs as recorded by the federal government's Drug Abuse Warning Network (DAWN).[6]

In 1978 and again in 1979, the House Select Committee on Narcotics Abuse and Control held public hearings on prescription drug abuse, and their conclusion was that these drugs were being overprescribed by physicians and diverted into the illegal market. A 1979 national survey conducted by the National Institute on Drug Abuse showed that the nonmedical use of prescription drugs was second only to the use of marijuana/hashish.

Many of the drugs that are addicting belong to that broad class of drugs called "painkillers." Americans spend over $1 billion a year on OTC painkillers alone. People are determined to use chemicals to avoid or alleviate pain. The nostrums of the great American medicine show during the 1800s brought more narcotics like opium and morphine into American homes than all the modern-day hard drug dealers combined. In 1900, for example, it has been estimated that 3,300,000 doses of opium were sold every month in the state of Vermont alone. That was enough to give every man, woman, and child in that state a continuous daily supply of one and one-half doses. Reports from this period suggested that the national population of those who became physically dependent on opium well exceeded 200,000. How could this have happened when people were partaking of such innocent-sounding concoctions as "Ayer's Cherry Pectoral," "Dover's Powder," "McMunn's Elixir of Opium," "Godfrey's Cordial," or "Mrs. Winslow's Soothing Syrup"? Their manufacturers made extraordinary claims for this wide assortment of compounds and elixirs, covering every malady from diarrhea to "women's troubles" to "consumption cures."

What was really going on was that people were either relieving pain getting high, or were "blissed out" (as with tranquilizers) by these opium-containing "medicines." Morphine was even used by some doctors to treat alcoholism. The result was that many of the alcoholics switched over and became morphine addicts.

In 1906 the Pure Food and Drug Act was passed. This act required that medicines containing opiates and certain other drugs had to say so on their labels, along with drug quantity and purity. But it wasn't until the passing of the Harrison Narcotics Act of 1914 that all opiates were removed from the open market and made available only through a doctor's prescription.

Analgesics are painkilling drugs. Opiates like morphine began the widespread use of such drugs over a hundred years ago. Many soldiers during the Civil War were treated with morphine and then spent many postwar years with a "medical addiction," that is, an unintentional addiction caused by the administration of the drug for pain relief. In order to be an ideal painkiller an analgesic drug would have to:

1. be potent enough to afford maximum pain relief;
2. be nonaddicting;
3. exhibit a minimum of side effects such as constipation, nausea, vomiting, and respiratory depression;
4. not cause tolerance to develop;
5. act promptly and over a long period of time with a minimum amount of sedation;
6. be relatively inexpensive.

One might ask whether the fact that opiates cause feelings of euphoria is a beneficial effect. It would certainly seem so, but part of our Puritan heritage is the Protestant prohibition against pleasure. Although pharmaceutical manufacturers are sparing no resources in the search for the ideal analgesic, it continues to elude them. Many products were once promoted as nonaddicting narcotics but usage over time inevitably led to physical and psychological dependency. Included among these drugs are heroin (which has no current medical usage in the United States), Demerol (meperidine), Dilaudid (hydromorphone), and the latest contestant, Talwin (pentazocine). When pentazocine was first introduced in 1967 it was believed that it came close to the ideal. However, it was soon learned that the drug can produce both physical and psychological dependence if used in large doses for an extended period of time, thus making it useful only for short-term management of pain.

Chronic pain is often a major feature in terminal illness. Recurring or persistent pain is most often accompanied by anxiety, depression, loss of appetite, and the inability to sleep. The hospice movement which began in England and spread to the United States has developed a compassionate and humanistic approach to pain management. In 1975 at St. Christopher's hospice in London an oral medication known as Brompton's Mixture provided patients with significant relief from the pain and distress associated with terminal cancer. Brompton's mixture, or "cocktail," consisted of:

diamorphine HCL	5–10 mg
cocaine	10 mg
alcohol (90%)	1.25 ml
syrup	2.5 ml
chloroform water to	10 ml

A phenothiazine was also given to potentiate, or boost, the effect of diamorphine (heroin), and to act as an antinausea drug and tranquilizer. Brompton's cocktail has been replaced in the United States by a morphine-alcohol solution commonly known as "hospice mix." This combination of ingredients is morphine sulfate in a 20 percent alcohol solution, to which flavoring agents and sugar are usually added. The side effect of sedation from the administration of morphine every four hours tends to disappear after a few days. Constipation can be treated with a combination of diet and stool softeners. This treatment can also be used at home in cases of similar life-threatening illness. (Consult your physician regarding the medical and legal aspects of such treatment.)

It is not only the narcotic or analgesic drugs that can cause any one of the three types of addiction. Let's consider two natural bodily functions: bowel movements and clear nasal passages. From time to time we all experience constipation. If you take a laxative you may come to depend upon that laxative to obtain normal bowel movements. Once this happens (and remember, there is no mood alteration or getting high with this kind of drug), you are in trouble. If constipation persists it may be because the constipation is a symptom of an underlying disorder and you should consult your doctor. When there is no pathological condition existing, it is better to find nonchemical ways to treat the problem of constipation—such as proper diet. The "rebound effect," which occurs when the desired state brought about by a drug leads to a dependency upon the drug, has been known to happen with nasal sprays as well. The spray clears up your nasal congestion for a while and then you find yourself stuffed up again or maybe feeling even worse, so it's back to the spray. This is a growing problem among cocaine sniffers, who use nasal sprays to deal with their chronically runny noses. It doesn't take long for the functional addiction to develop. Both of these are examples of functional addictions and rarely are conceived of as drug dependencies. But they are addictions just as real as the psychological and physical ones.

There are OTCs that can lead to physical dependencies and worse. The FDA has been warning people about a painkiller called phenacetin (acetophenetidin) since 1977, stating that it "is not safe for OTC use because of the high potential for abuse, the high potential for harm to the kidney . . . and the lack of compensating benefits of the drug." The FDA has concluded that this drug has high abuse potential, giving the user a slight euphoric feeling along with mild stimulation. But it's still on the market in a variety of OTCs. According to the 1982 *Physicians' Desk Reference,* the following medications still contain phenacetin:

A.P.C. tablets	Emprazil-C tablets
A.P.C. with Butalbital	Fiorinal
A.P.C. with Codeine	Fiorinal with Codeine
Apectol tablets	SK-65 Compound Capsules
Butalbital with APC tablets	Soma Compound
Emprazil tablets	Soma Compound with Codeine

Check the label on *all* OTCs to see if they contain this drug as well.

There are drugs like diazepam (Valium) which can be physically or psychologically addictive or both. Some physicians are easily manipulated by "street wise" drug users for these types of drugs. Hypnotic sedatives like Quaalude, Parest, and Sopor are popular with these manipulators. Large doses of these cause physical and psychological dependency. One has to take care with cross-addicting drugs as well. For example, a person who takes barbiturates and also drinks alcohol, both in subaddicting amounts, may find himself developing a tolerance, as both are sedatives with very similar chemical actions.

Because so many drugs have side effects, adverse reactions, contraindications, addiction potential, and the like, it has become very important to know as much as possible about the drugs we take. The drug manufacturers and the doctors don't seem to want us to know too much about the drugs they produce and prescribe. Why else are they fighting the institution of patient package inserts, and why else is the FDA dragging its feet on this issue? Like so many issues involving drugs, there are two sides to the coin. You already know the "down side" about how patients are treated as ignorant children by drug companies and many doctors. The other side of the coin, at least from the doctor's point of view, is that there really are patients who, if told about a certain potential drug effect, will be certain to experience that effect. People are very open to suggestion, especially when they are sick, and doctors are afraid that telling us what might happen when we take a drug, particularly side effects and adverse reactions, will guarantee that it will happen. Perhaps many of us deserve to be viewed this way by our doctors. By abdicating personal responsibility for drug taking and placing it all in the hands of someone we perceive as being the right hand of God, we have brought this grief down on our own heads. When we take back this personal responsibility, then we can say to the doctor, "I want to know everything that is important in making a benefit/risk decision about this drug!" And that includes information about habit-forming drugs. We must know whether or not medicines contain ingredients that risk any of the three types of drug addiction. This has implications for:

- deciding whether or not to take the drug.
- avoiding the addictive potential.
- respecting the importance of taking it only as prescribed.
- planning for discontinuation of the drug so that none of its potential for dependence and tolerance, and therefore withdrawal syndrome effects, are realized.
- checking out your desire to use this drug for purposes other than it was intended.
- avoiding tolerance and the need for escalating doses.

Many people have become addicted to OTC and prescription medications through ignorance. Educate yourself and know what you are taking!

ALTERNATIVES

As you have just read, all is not well in our modern world of standard medicine. After reading about the many risks and dangers involved in contemporary drug therapy, it is only natural for the question to arise, Are there alternatives? The answer is yes, but you must be willing to greatly expand your awareness of approaches that fall outside of standard medicine. Once you have done this you are in a far better position to choose from a broader range of remedies. The central idea is to view "traditional" and "contemporary" methods of healing not as antagonistic, but rather as points along a broad continuum of possible remedies. I commend to you the holistic view as an organizing principle around which to make these important choices. Here I mean that holistic medicine is a model rather than just a series of techniques that define its practice. Here are the elements that are central to this model.[7]

1. Holistic medicine addresses itself to the physical, mental, and spiritual aspects of those who come for care.

211

2. Although it appreciates the predictive value of data which are based on statistical models, holistic medicine emphasizes each patient's genetic, biological, and psychosocial uniqueness as well as the importance of tailoring treatment to meet each individual's needs.

3. A holistic approach to medicine and health care includes understanding and treating people in the context of their culture, their family, and their community.

4. Holistic medicine views health as a positive state, not as the absence of disease.

5. Holistic medicine emphasizes the responsibility of each individual for his or her health.

6. Holistic medicine emphasizes the promotion of health and the prevention of disease.

7. Holistic medicine uses therapeutic approaches that mobilize the individual's innate capacity for self-healing.

8. Though none would deny the occasional necessity for swift and authoritative medical or surgical intervention, the emphasis in holistic medicine is on helping people to understand and to help themselves, on education and self-care rather than treatment and dependence.

9. Holistic medicine makes use of a variety of diagnostic methods and systems in addition to and sometimes in place of the standard laboratory examinations.

10. Physical contact between practitioner and patient is an important element of holistic medicine.

11. Good health depends on good nutrition and regular exercise.

12. Holistic medicine includes an appreciation of and attention to sensuousness and sexuality.

13. Holistic medicine views illness as an opportunity for discovery as well as misfortune.

14. Holism includes an appreciation of the quality of life in each of its stages and an interest in improving it as

well as acknowledgment of the illnesses that are common to it.

15. Holistic medicine emphasizes the potential therapeutic value of the setting in which health care takes place.

16. An understanding of and a commitment to change those social and economic conditions that perpetuate ill health are as much a part of holistic medicine as its emphasis on individual responsibility.

17. Holistic medicine transforms its practitioners as well as its patients.

The kind of active partnership between patient/consumer and practitioner implied in this model makes you far more responsible for your own state of health and well-being. To participate in this model means giving up the notion of "instant" relief and dependence on practitioners as the sole dispensers of relief and comfort. The good news is that a willingness to embrace this model can often mean a real decrease in reliance on drug therapies for many maladies. It means moving from being the passive recipient of pills and elixirs to being the active promoter of your own relatively drug-free health. Listed below are some of the techniques and therapies which have become an active part of holistic medical practice in the United States and other countries.

Biofeedback: With the aid of electronically enhanced biological feedback, physiological mechanisms, previously believed to be outside of voluntary control, can be controlled by the individual after brief training periods. Biofeedback has positive effects on such problems as tension headaches, migraine, essential hypertension, insomnia, Raynaud's disease, sinus, tachycardia, bronchial asthma, functional colitis, stuttering, urinary retention, sexual dysfunctions, drug abuse, hyperactivity, anxiety, and phobias.

Autogenic Training: A highly systematized technique designed to generate a state of psychophysiological relaxation, the opposite of the state of stress. Specific practices and exercises are taught that allow the individual to achieve a state of deep relaxation, enabling the body and mind to carry out their own recuperative and healing processes.

Meditation: Meditation is a whole family of techniques that have in common a conscious attempt to focus attention. It is used to achieve altered states of consciousness and as a system of self-regulation. It can induce powerful subjective changes in one's view of one's self, of nature, and of other people. It can lead to altered states similar to those brought about by hypnosis and deep muscle relaxation exercises.

Hypnosis: Hypnosis may be many things but is generally agreed upon as some sort of altered awareness and behavior as compared with the presumably normal awake state. It can be used as posthypnotic suggestion to directly relieve symptoms and to override any unconscious resistance, or as a medium for substituting good physical responses for disturbed ones, and can gain access to selective memory to reveal cause-and-effect relationships in physical and emotional problems. It is used to help manage pain, as a technique of anesthesia, in obstetrics and gynecology, and as a means of communicating with unconscious or critically ill patients.

Chiropractic: Chiropractic involves manipulation of the spine and joints and views the nervous system as the crucial element in proper bodily functioning. Recently chiropractors have begun to include diet and exercise regimens and healing modalities such as acupuncture, massage, and homeopathy. Chiropractic is seen as an alternative to surgical and pharmacologic remedies. As research efforts increase, more objective evidence of the value and importance of alteration in musculoskeletal structures to bodily functioning may be demonstrated. For the moment, most testimonials are individual. Most of you know someone who swears by their chiropractor.

Acupuncture: Chinese medicine seeks to maintain or restore a balance between yang and yin much as our concept of homeostasis, which refers to a balance of opposite forces to insure proper functioning of physiological systems. Tiny hair-thin needles are painlessly inserted and removed, and while in place they create a tingling or heavy sensation. Modern research shows that acupuncture is most effective as an alternative to analgesic drugs in the management of certain kinds of pain: musculoskeletal pain, muscle contraction, migraine headaches, and various neuralgias. It is used as an alternative to surgical or pharmacologic management of pain and for some patients is an extremely effective technique.

Homeopathic Medicine: From the Greek *homois,* meaning similar, and *pathos,* meaning suffering or sickness. The basic law of homeopathy is based on the law of similars, or "like is cured by like." The law of similars states that a remedy or medicine can cure a disease if it produces in a healthy person symptoms similar to that of the disease. This stimulates the body's own healing powers. Homeopaths do not prescribe combination drugs, preferring to work with one symptom and one medicine at a time. They also stress minimum dosage. They also believe that much chronic disease is due to the incorrect treatment of prior acute illness, leading to its suppression and eventual emergence in a chronic form.

There are other techniques and therapies too numerous to describe here, such as herbalism, natural medicine (naturopathy), exercise, food and nutrition, light and sound in health, psychic healing, touch, etc. For further readings on the subject consult the bibliography.

CHAPTER FIVE

Getting High

In this chapter we will take a look at the risks and benefits that accompany the use of pleasure drugs. You may hear people refer to them by a variety of names—recreational, pleasure, street, leisure, good times drugs. They all refer to the assortment of drugs that are used in the pursuit of pleasurable states. Regardless of what drug we are talking about—a martini, a fine wine, a cold beer, a joint (marijuana cigarette), a line of cocaine, a handful of ludes (methaqualone)—the end result of drug use is the same: a change in our mood and consciousness. Is the desire to alter consciousness periodically an innate, normal drive analagous to hunger or the sex drive? Seventy percent of adult America drinks alcoholic beverages; over 15 million people have tried cocaine; over 40 million people have tried marijuana and some 12 million use it regularly; and so it goes for many other drugs as well. The National Institute on Drug Abuse recently estimated that Americans spend at least $120 billion a year on controlled substances and their consequences.

DON'T PUT IT INTO YOUR SYSTEM UNLESS YOU KNOW WHAT IT'LL DO TO YOU

Remember when you were a little kid and your mother warned about what could happen if you placed foreign objects in your mouth? She was concerned about your health and did not want you to get sick. The same warning still holds true today and can easily be applied to drug usage. But it isn't just your mouth that you need to exercise caution about. There are many ways to take drugs: you can inject them into your body (skin popping just under the surface or mainlining, heading straight for a vein); you can smoke them (using rolling papers, bongs, carburetors, pipes, and other smoking paraphernalia); you can ingest them through the mucous membranes of your nose (sniffing and snorting); you can drink them (and not just alcohol: people who are into reggae music and the Jamaican culture enjoy drinking concoctions made with cannabis extracts); and you can eat them (anything from hash brownies to psychedelic mushrooms like peyote and psilocybin). Pill takers, particularly fans of barbiturates and hypnotics like Quaaludes (methaqualone), often speak of "eating" their pills. There are a lot of ways to get high.

How do you really know what you are putting into your system? Let's say you are at a party and drugs are offered. This is the time to remember your mother's warning. Once you are high, it may be too late. Everybody is so busy being hip, bragging about their "reliable" connections and the good "shit" that they were able to "cop."

When you go into a liquor store or supermarket and purchase a bottle of spirits or wine or beer, you believe you are getting what it says on the label, including type of spirits and alcohol content. You assume purity and quantity of dose because your experience has taught you that these things are uniform from purchase to purchase. The same holds true, in general, for prescription drugs and over-the-counter medications. But have you ever stopped to consider what really is in alcoholic drinks? One researcher, Hebe B. Greizerstein, of the New York State Division of Alcoholism and Alcohol Abuse, has found that, along with the principal active ingredient, ethanol, most alcoholic beverages contain such items as lead, iron, cobalt, histamines, tannins, phenols, and trace amounts of a large number of other organic and inorganic compounds.[1] The Center for Science in the Public Interest claims that over a million people may be allergic to substances in beer, wine, and liquor. They cite, as one example, the common preservative sulfur dioxide as causing allergic reactions, and further claim that yellow dye no. 5, allowed in beer and spirits, has brought problems to "tens of thousands" of aspirin-sensitive people. The beverage industry has fought against labeling requirements, claiming they are expensive and unnecessary, and that consumers would not understand them. Is it safe to assume these ingredients carry no health risks? One class of chemical compounds added to alcoholic beverages, called cogeners, are already suspected of being largely responsible for variety in the severity of hangovers. The answer to this question should probably be the same as the cautions regarding marijuana use, namely that in the absence of conclusive scientific evidence, if you must drink alcohol or smoke grass, judicious moderation and an alertness to new discoveries are in order. In the interim it would certainly be helpful to consumers in calculating risks and benefits of alcoholic beverage consumption if the products carried labels that disclose all the ingredients.

Having considered alcohol products that you had previously taken for granted, consider the fact that once you step into the world of illicit or pleasure drugs, all bets are off concerning acts of faith! This same act of faith applied to drugs bought "on the street" can lead to serious trouble. The products are not labeled, there are no assurances of quality control, many substances resemble each other in color and consistency, price varies greatly, and the seller does not have to comply with any licensing or regulatory requirements. To put it mildly, appearances can be very deceptive, and you won't find any warnings from the surgeon general's office either. And yet millions of people are making drug-taking an act of faith every day. Very few stop to consider the psychology of drug taking as an act of faith.

In the partying situation we tend to assume that:

- the drug is what people say it is;
- our friends and acquaintances would not give us anything harmful;
- if we are told this is "good stuff," there is no need to question it;
- the dose is reliable;
- we are going to get high in ways we have previously experienced.

Taking these kinds of things for granted has gotten people into serious trouble.

It is much safer to ask questions than to make this act of faith. Check it out! Be skeptical. Don't let anyone else assume your responsibility for something that you are going to put into your body. Ask questions about the drugs you are offered, and if you don't like the tone or content of the answers, *don't take the drug!* Remember, if you decide to take the drug you must be prepared to live with the consequences, good and bad.

Jim's story

Jim always thought of himself as a pretty hip drug user. He had never been beat in a drug deal, and always got what he paid for. He prided himself on his ability to score good stuff and enjoyed turning on his friends. When his usual marijuana connection got busted he heard about a new one from a "friend." He bought a dime bag ($10) of what he was told was high-quality grass and proceeded to share it with three friends. They all smoked, expecting to get a nice marijuana high. Within twenty minutes two of his friends were acting very weird and Jim was starting to experience feelings of paranoia. Realizing that something was terribly wrong, they had the good sense to go to a hospital emergency room. One of his friends became violent and had to be restrained. Fortunately, the doctor in the ER knew his street drugs. The boys had smoked some very low-grade grass which had been laced with angel dust (PCP or phencyclidine), a volatile and powerful animal tranquilizer with hallucinatory effects. Neither Jim nor his friends thought he was very hip after that experience.

Phencyclidine (PCP, hog, angel dust) was formerly used to sedate large animals like jungle cats and elephants, but it made them so agitated and disoriented before putting them under that it has been abandoned by veterinarians. Kids picked up on it as a drug which causes a strong high and certain psychedelic effects (similar to marijuana). However, it carries some awesome unwanted side effects like severe disorientation, paranoia, violent behavior, depression, and confusion, so that its risks far outweigh any apparent user benefits. It rarely affects the same person the same way upon subsequent use and is therefore very unpredictable. It's a real bummer and should be avoided altogether. Take a lesson from Jim and his friends. This is one of those "I dare you to try it" drugs. Stay away from it!

Drug dealing is a very lucrative and a virtually uncontrollable business. Unscrupulous dealers find plenty of ways to cut corners and increase profits—all at your expense. Here are some examples of how they do it.

Ways to Get Beat in the Illicit Drug Market

What it's supposed to be	What it often turns out to be
High-grade marijuana	Low-grade (very little THC and other mind-altering ingredients)
	Oregano (sometimes laced with PCP)
	A mixture of a small amount of high-grade grass with a lot of low-grade stuff
Dexedrin, Eskabarb, Dalmane, Valium	Mild stimulants like ephedrin, caffeine, phenylpropanolamine, called "look-alike" drugs; sold in

What it's supposed to be	What it often turns out to be
	health stores and on the street. Danger is that you get a bogus reaction and are in trouble when you take the real thing because it's much stronger (false sense of being able to handle the drugs).
Amphetamines	Caffeine. You'll get a fraction of the lift at top-market prices.
Methaqualone (ludes)	Valium or phenobarbital (both very dangerous at high dose levels).
Cocaine	You get very little or no coke. Coke is cut with lactose (milk sugar), powered milk, Epsom salts, caffeine, talcum powder, sucrose, glucose, quinine, strychnine, aspirin, vitamins, cornstarch, menita, inositol, mannitol, and flour.
	You get coke substitutes like lidocaine, procaine, benzocaine, and tetracaine, which can collapse blood vessels, reduce heart muscle strength, and cause low blood pressure. A person who can handle coke could go into shock if he is allergic to coke substitutes.
Heroin	Low doses (1% to 4%) cut with a lot of quinine or milk sugar.
Assorted pills in capsule form	Dealer removes active ingredients and substitutes cheaper and sometimes dangerous ingredients.

Amphetamines are stimulant drugs which have been used by medicine for appetite suppression, abnormal hyperactivity disorders, and narcolepsy (sleep disorder). Picked up by the drug scene because of their boost to psychic and physical energy levels, they became the object of one of the few street prevention programs ever launched in this country. "Speed Kills" buttons were found in the East Village and the Haight-Ashbury areas during the late 1960s. Speed is making a comeback, but most of the stuff you buy on the street is not the genuine article. Dr. John Morgan reported in the *Journal of Psychoactive Drugs* that 90 percent of the street speed is look-alikes containing caffeine, phenylpropanolamine (a nasal decongestant and appetite suppressant), and ephedrine (a decongestant).[2] These clever look-alikes resemble the real thing, but actually give you very little bang for the buck and can be downright dangerous because of additives and impurities.

Methaqualone (Quaalude, Sopor, Parest) is a hypnotic (sleep inducer). Drug scene people like the alcohol-like high and tout the drug as giving a good "body high" somewhat like an aphrodisiac. In the case of ludes the unscrupulous dealer has several ways to cheat the consumer. It is rare to find the genuine article on the street. The counterfeits are referred to as bootlegs; the biggest item in this category is the Lemmon 714 (Lemmon manufactures legitimate Quaalude). The bootleg looks like the real McCoy, right down to the scoring and crispy edges. Sometimes these bootlegs are not made from raw methaqualone. Valium is substituted in high doses, leading to nasty and dangerous highs with vomiting and even the danger of coma, usually followed by a two-day hangover. The other common substitute is phenobarbital, which is a slow-acting, long-lasting barbiturate. Because it takes longer to experience the high than with real ludes, the user may take another. This is extremely dangerous because one lude-size dose of phenobarbital is greater than the therapeutic dose for a twenty-four-hour period; two is greater than the minimum lethal dose. Phenobarbital is very dangerous when mixed with alcohol because both are sedatives and the effects are additive.

Once you have decided to take a drug, it is a good idea to

titrate the dose in direct proportion to the information available about purity and dose. Titration is the chemist's process for determining the concentration of a substance in solution. The layman's version of this is as follows: the less you know about a drug, the more caution you want to exercise when taking it. By first taking a small amount and then waiting to experience the actual effects, you can save yourself some unwanted effects or at least minimize bad ones. Once you feel comfortable with what is actually happening to you, then you may opt to take a little more and again see how it actually works on your body and mind. Don't be a pig—it could lead to a real bad trip. You can also lose some of the more subtle effects of the drug. What's the hurry? There is one major caution here: many drugs alter the way in which we perceive the passage of time. Use a clock or watch, not your subjective senses (which are now altered), to check the time. You may wish to titrate known doses to make the effects last a little longer and to avoid the building-up of a tolerance to the drug (needing more to get the original effect) (this is how addiction begins). This "take a little and wait" approach is used by seasoned pleasure seekers.

This caution can save your life, particularly when mixing drugs. The following story shows what can happen, even to street-wise drug users, when perceptions are altered by drugs.

Dino's Story

Dino did drugs between the ages of fourteen and eighteen. His life was out of control, and he spent two years in a drug-free residential treatment program to do some growing up. Five years out of treatment, he slipped back into heroin addiction. He began using methadone he purchased in the street to slowly detoxify himself from the heroin. Withdrawal from opiates is often accompanied by sleep disturbance. After forty-eight hours of not sleeping, Dino added one more element to his home remedy. He got hold of some barbiturates to help him to sleep, but he had absolutely no experience with this type of drug (preferring opiates and hallucinogens). He took two "goofballs" (phenobarbital), and after what he thought was one hour (actually only ten minutes), he took two more. The next thing I knew, Dino had me on the phone; he was very drowsy but in a definite state of confusion and panic. I used every tactic I could think of (including having him put an ice pack on his testicles) to keep him walking and talking, while I called the emergency squad on the other phone. He was okay, but the ambulance driver told me that if he had fallen asleep he would probably never have regained consciousness.

People like to share drugs, and this means that they will also share the various equipment used to get high. Passing joints, pipes, bongs, hookahs (water pipes), carburetors, and other smoking apparatus is quite common. However, so are colds, flu, and herpes (simplex and not so simplex). The same holds true for devices used to sniff cocaine, which are usually inserted into one's nostrils. Dirty needles transmit hepatitis and other communicable diseases. Air bubbles in syringes can kill you. Sharing equipment is another act of faith that can get you in trouble. No one's naked eye can see the microbes that can cause the trouble. Remember that we are in the midst of a venereal disease epidemic and some really nice hip people are transmitting these diseases through an act of love! The same cautions apply to the "loving sharing" of drugs. So keep your act clean, exercise a little caution, and your drug experiences won't cost you.

COCAINE—THE HIGH PRICE OF GETTING HIGH

Cocaine is an alkaloid derived from the leaves of the *Erythroxylon coca* (a shrub which is cultivated in, among other places, Peru, Chile, Bolivia, and Mexico). It starts as a residue extracted from the leaves ($200 to $300 a pound), and when refined and cut with various products costs anywhere from $1800 to $2500 per ounce (for high-quality, relatively pure coke). Current street prices put the final adulterated product (12 percent cocaine) at about $100 to $150 per gram (the amount most commonly purchased by users). The American public used to have easy and legal access to cocaine in the form of such innocent-sounding nostrums as "Agnew's Powder," "Anglo-American Catarrh Powder," and "Ryno's Hay Fever and Catarrh Remedy." Many of what we now call over-the-counter (OTC) drugs contained cocaine and sold like hotcakes between the 1890s and 1914, the year the Harrison Narcotics Act was passed. Although cocaine is a stimulant drug with no narcotic features, in 1922 Congress prohibited most importation of coca leaves and officially defined it as a narcotic (a designation that still applies today). Cocaine used to be an ingredient in the original Coca-Cola formula (dropped in 1903) and was advertised "to cure your headache" and "relieve fatigue" for only 5 cents. Émile Gautier's Vin Mariani was celebrated by many famous people during that same time. Popes Leo XIII and Pius X, Sarah Bernhardt, Émile Zola, Jules Verne, and H. G. Wells all endorsed this rather plebeian wine which contained a tiny proportion of coca extract. Bernhardt said, "Vin Mariani is indispensable to dramatic and lyric artists. I would be unable to go on without it." Enrico Caruso stated of Vin Mariani, "I found it excellent for the voice. It gives particular energy to the artist when fatigued." It sold well in Europe and to a lesser extent in America before Gautier's death and the Harrison Act put it out of business. The most famous of cocaine's proponents was a Viennese neurologist named Sigmund Freud. In writing of his personal experiences with the drug to his fiancée, Martha Bernays, Freud stated:

> Woe to you, my Princess, when I come. I will kiss you quite red and feed you till you are plump. And if you are froward you shall see who is the stronger, a gentle little girl who doesn't eat enough or a big wild man who has cocaine in his body. In my last severe depression I took coca again and a small dose lifted me to the heights in a wonderful fashion. I am now busy collecting the literature for a song of praise to this magical substance.[3]

Sounds like great stuff when you read these accounts! Here is a more up-to-date account of what can happen when you play with cocaine.

Arthur's story

I started out snorting a little in my friends' homes. It hit me immediately what a nice drug I had discovered. Sure it cost a lot of money but I was always into showing off anyway. Addicting? I thought not—after all, this wasn't heroin or speed. So I began buying it by the gram at first and then by the ounce, telling myself I was actually saving money by buying it in larger quantities. I was able to make love longer, rap longer, and everything was so crystal clear and beautiful. At first I could stay high for about fifteen or twenty minutes after a few blows [snorts], but later on I would only stay up for about ten minutes. The trips got shorter and the drug bills got higher. What I did not realize is that I was becoming obsessed with coke. I reached the point where all I wanted to do was get high. People were always hitting on me for coke or money to buy coke. I experienced some real bad depressions after coming down so I dedicated my life to staying "up." People started telling me that I was acting increasingly paranoid and weird but I just said "that's the drug" and kept right on going. At the point at which I finally stopped I was spending about $4,000 a month on coke and had completely lost my perspective on my work, my friends, sex, everything!

Cocaine is not physically addicting, but psychological dependency (the desire to bring about this altered state repeatedly) is very real. This psychic dependency stems from the drug's powerful euphoric reaction. Even laboratory animals love it. One report states that rats would press a bar 250 times to obtain caffeine, 4000 consecutive times to obtain heroin, and 10,000 times in a row to obtain cocaine. That's a pretty powerful positive reinforcer. Richard Pryor, who knows how enticing the drug can be, stated in his film *Live on the Sunset Strip:* "You've been doing it more than two weeks—you're a junkie. You won't be able to stop." Pryor reportedly almost burned to death as a result of freebasing cocaine. Freebasing is a method of processing cocaine hydrochloride down to its most powerful essence and then smoking it;

the ether used in the process is highly flammable. Most users snort it sharply up into their nostrils using rolled bills, straws, or coke spoons. Some people inject it into their veins. This method of administration leads to a euphoric "rush" and feelings of elation which have often been compared to a sexual orgasm (this is probably due to the greater amount taken into the body this way), but it causes a loss of subtle effects, and the euphoria is shorter-lived. Therefore the peak experience and the "comedown" occur more rapidly. The addiction liability increases as the user moves from snorting to freebasing to injection. Most researchers do not report a tolerance effect with cocaine, but more and more chronic users are reporting that the trips on coke get shorter and less intense, requiring larger quantities of purer dose to achieve the original euphoric effect. This may be a "temporary tolerance," which is experienced only by chronic users and not by periodic pleasure seekers. Some users mix the coke with heroin (called a speedball) to prolong the pleasant effects and produce a "roller coaster effect." The catch is that the roller coaster can make you feel "like you're tearing your body in half." This is how John Belushi is reported to have ended his life. It's hard to know, as Belushi was reported to have been into coke, heroin, and alcohol. Cocaine may potentiate the lethal nature of heroin.

There is no doubt that cocaine is increasing in popularity. Over 15 million people have used it in the United States, and it has made the cover of *Time* magazine. Although the number of primary cocaine abusers is low (about 2 percent) in federally funded drug treatment programs, the number has tripled in the past several years. Cocaine-related deaths are relatively few in number (19.1 deaths per 10,000 medical-examiner reports), but they have also been reported on the increase (up from 4.5 deaths per 10,000). One of the main problems with drug-related statistics is that we don't know how many such deaths went undetected because of ignorance or because the drug was metabolized completely before death (this takes about six hours for coke). Doctors also often fail to list drugs or alcohol as the cause to save the family any "embarassment."

One of the reasons for cocaine's popularity is its purported role as an aphrodisiac. Some users claim it actually causes sexual arousal, while others state that it enhances the sexual experience. Since cocaine is a topical anesthetic (it can deaden sensation), it has been rubbed on the head of the penis or on the clitoris to prolong intercourse. Many of coke's sexual claims are dose-related (use too much and you blow it). With doses of a gram or less per day, coke may enhance sexuality, delay ejaculation, and produce more intense and satisfying orgasms. At higher doses users often report a decreased interest in sexuality. In fact, sex can't compete with coke at higher levels of regular use.

So why a special caution about cocaine? There are several reasons. The first is that people con themselves into believing that coke is "safe" and nonaddicting and refuse to exercise the respect the drug should command from everyone. The euphoric effects of the drug are powerfully reinforcing, and users want to repeat the experience again and again. The gradual building up of psychic dependence leading to a compulsion is slow and insidious. People who have found that marijuana has caused them no problems believe that they will have the same experience with coke. Drugs are like coins—they have two sides. If coke has a side that is a powerful reinforcer, it also has its dark side. If you feel increased mental and physical strength while using coke, how might you feel when the coke wears off? You are borrowing future energy and, like a bank loan, it has to be paid back. You feel let down, ordinary, maybe a little depressed. Either you let this feeling pass or you decide to get back up, which means you have to do some more coke. This is how the craving for the drug can insidiously creep into your life. You like the high so much that everything else feels like a "low." If you are freebasing, mainlining, or snorting regularly (daily), you run the risk of "crashing." This crashing is somewhat comparable to what happens after a speed "run" (many hours or even days of shooting amphetamines). Crashing involves profound feelings of the opposite of euphoria—dysphoria. One way to describe dysphoria is as the inability to create and hold good feelings. As chronic use increases and/or dosage goes up, the user runs the risk of going

beyond dysphoria into a full-blown cocaine psychosis with paranoid delusions and hallucinations. The main reaction to the stopping of coke use is a feeling of depression. This reactive depression
(in reaction to the absence of the drug) is accompanied by intense
craving, represented by an overpowering compulsion to continue
using the drug.

Another problem associated with cocaine is its price. It's the
status drug—the one that lets everybody know you are a person
of means. In the drug scene it's the ultimate ego trip. If you
have enough to turn on your friends, you get the oohs and aahs
that go with all conspicuous consumption (until you run out of
coke). Prices keep going up (supply and demand) and potency
generally goes down (more adulterant, less coke). People who
become psychologically dependent upon the drug spend incredible
amounts of money on it. When you factor it out, it comes to
something on the order of about $200 per hour of being
high. Coke becomes more important than anything else. In 1980
alone street sales of cocaine reached an estimated $30 billion.

Cocaine, like many other stimulants including caffeine, acts
as an appetite supressant. But before you run out to score some
coke as a diet aid, remember the price, both in dollars and in
possible problems. Cocaine is a powerful seducer. Your money,
your sex life, your friendships, your job—all may be replaced
by that fine white powder. This is one drug that means business.

Less is known about the physical problems. One often hears
reports of heavy users having nasal problems. However, the number of users suffering the worst of these problems—the perforation
of the nasal septum (the membrane dividing the two halves of
the nose)—is rare but on the increase. The major adverse physical
reactions involving cocaine are reported to be inflammation of
the nasal mucosa, nasal sores, and nasal bleeding. These problems
are caused by particles of the drug that become lodged in the
small hair follicles of the nose. If they get caught in the sinus
cavities, they can cause headaches and congestion. This leads
to the characteristic runny nose seen in many regular coke users.
To avoid this, users chop up the larger flakes or crystals with
a razor blade to make it into as fine a powder as possible (more

absorption of coke and fewer particles to clog). Users will also "snort" water or nasal sprays to keep the mucosa clear of particles. Again, as cocaine is a topical anesthetic it causes feelings of numbness in the nose, throat, and sinuses. Freebasing is probably dangerous to the respiratory system because it constricts the blood vessels of the lungs. Cocaine users who inject the drug run all the risks that heroin addicts, speed freaks, and all so-called needle freaks (people who do drugs with syringes) run. These include abscesses and sores, overdosing, hepatitis, tetanus, pneumonia, and lung abscesses.

Addiction can be defined as having three elements: (1) compulsion (repetitive urge), (2) negative consequences, and (3) loss of control (the drug takes over). This definition can help you to see that people can get "strung out" on coke just as with many other drugs. You must weigh the risks and the benefits. Any drug that can promise as much pleasure and excitement as cocaine requires thoughtfulness and caution when used. If you must do coke:

- do it infrequently;
- don't mess with needles;
- take proper care of your nose;
- make sure you can afford it;
- remember that it's a felony bust if you get caught;
- remember it can lead to heavy-duty psychic dependence;
- remember it can lift you up real high and set you down hard;
- don't freebase—it's a much quicker route to dependency;
- make sure it's the "real thing" and not an adulterant or substitute.

The National Institute on Drug Abuse has found no health problems associated with "recreational use" defined as one to two grams a week or less taken nasally. "Most coke users don't get into trouble," says Dr. Robert C. Peterson, NIDA's director of research. "Even regular users probably just snort up on weekends like in Woody Allen movies." Sticking to this pattern of use requires vigilance and self honesty on the part of the user or the dangers listed above will become part of your cocaine experience.

The use of cocaine has become so pervasive in areas of the country like Hollywood, California, that new treatment approaches are springing up to meet the problem. Modeled after Alcoholics Anonymous, Pills Anonymous, and Smoke Enders, programs vary in cost and effectiveness. "Coke Enders" meets at Wilbur Hot Springs Health Sanctuary, a health farm in Williams, north of San Francisco. Another program is run by the Beverly Glen Hospital in Los Angeles. One group that meets on the West Coast boasts so many celebrities that one person says, "On a good night it's like walking in Ma Maison [a prominent Beverly Hills restaurant] or Elaine's." Most people attempting to stop the compulsive use of cocaine will require a great deal of group support to achieve their goal. This is particularly true when they develop a dual addiction, to alcohol or other sedatives used to ease the "crashing" after a coke run. These people must learn to be abstinent from both the uppers and the downers.

LUDES

Methaqualone was introduced in 1965 as a sedative-hypnotic (it will calm you and induce sleep) that was touted as being safer and less addicting than barbiturates (Seconal, Tuinal, Nembutal, Butisol, Amytal). It is manufactured in the United States as Parest (Parke-Davis), Quaalude (Lemmon), and Sopor (Arnar-Stone). Some of the street names for methaqualone are ludes, love drug, Qs, quas, quads, 714s, sopers, wallbangers, and disco biscuits. Ludes were intended to provide relief of mild to moderate anxiety or tension (sedative effect), and at higher doses taken at bedtime to relieve insomnia (hypnotic effect). Some of the side effects are lightheadedness in the upright position, weakness, and unsteadiness in stance and gait. Users are warned by doctors prescribing methaqualone not to take it for more than three months continuously. Ludes took off like a rocket, becoming the sixth most frequently prescribed drug in this country. In some sections of the country "lude doctors" began to prescribe the drug for anyone with vague complaints of being tense or suffering from sleeplessness (and willing to pay the price of an office visit, ranging anywhere from $25 to $150). Lude users exchange names of these doctors and end up with multiple prescriptions, usually selling many of the pills for $8 to $10 apiece. One of my patients in New York City tells the following story:

> It's getting real hard to cop authentic ludes on the street. So your best bet is to tie into two or three lude docs. All you have to do is talk about how uptight you are and how you can't sleep, and you've got yourself a prescription— no other questions asked. This way you get a legal script, go to your local pharmacy, get your pills, and you're in business. I usually keep a few bottles for myself and sell the rest at $9 apiece.

Remember the warning about adulterants? The Drug Enforcement Administration found a shipment of raw methaqualone in Florida in April 1982 that could have given hepatitis to thousands. Ludes are rarely prescribed by conscientious doctors. A sharp drop has been reported in prescriptions by New York doctors, and the decline has been attributed to prosecutions of "stress-relief centers" which used licensed physicians for the mass prescribing of the drug. The drop was also aided by better controls on its distribution by the manufacturers.

You may have noticed that ludes are called the "love drug." That's because part of the lore on ludes is that they are the aphrodisiac-of-choice for people who are into sex and drugs. *High Times* magazine said that "methaqualone did for seduction what McDonald's did for hamburgers." One or two ludes make the user feel a tingling relaxation of the body's muscles, a warm feeling, a sense of disinhibition and recklessness, and a flaring of sexual desire. It induces feelings of closeness and intimacy between relative strangers and artificially transposes a mild attraction into a "deep understanding." That certainly explains why someone might be tempted to drop a few pills. But this drug carries with it some real dangers that fans are not likely to tell you about. There is real addiction liability—both physical and psychological. After a couple of weeks of steady use, inexperienced users find themselves eating ludes like candy. Tolerance sets in very quickly and you need more and more to get the original desired effect. This leads the user to believe that the drug is relatively safe. But with escalating use, the difference between a dose that can get you high and one that can kill you gets smaller and smaller. More than ten tablets and you can suffer a fatal overdose.

Ludes in combination with alcohol can produce stupor, coma, and respiratory depression. This is called "luding out." The main danger of luding out is that methaqualone (like many tranquilizers) suppresses the gag reflex. A passed-out person who vomits may breathe in the vomit, leading to brain damage or death from oxygen loss.

Watching someone who is really stoned on ludes is like watching a drunk. Large doses cause a numbness in the arms, neck, and skull; minor injuries will not be felt until the drug wears off. Flaccid arms and spastic legs are not uncommon, and the person is quite disoriented. Speech is slurred and often incoherent. Suddenly stopping the drug can lead to withdrawal with convulsions. All detoxification should be done in a hospital setting. Ludes can also lead to some nasty hangovers, particularly when combined with alcohol. As sedatives usually mess up sexual performance, the so-called aphrodisiac effect is probably nothing more than the releasing of inhibitions (similar to the effect of relatively small amounts of alcohol). Once you have experienced "better sex" with ludes, you run the risk of not striving for sexual enjoyment without the drug. So if you must use this risky drug you are well advised to use it infrequently and in small amounts.

HEROIN

The word "heroin" derived from the German word *heroisch*, which means heroic or powerful. The drug is aptly named, because as one junkie I know puts it: "Man, it's the greatest feeling

233

in the world 'cause it's the feeling of nonfeeling. Nothing gets through—no physical pain and no mental pain. The biggest loser feels like a winner when he's high on smack." There are basically three ways to use heroin: snort it like cocaine; "skin-pop" it by injecting it just under the surface of the skin (like an allergist's scratch test); "mainline" it by injecting it right into a vein. Middle-class people not driven to blotting out the harsh realities of daily life at the bottom of the social heap have tended to shy away from needle drugs like heroin and methamphetamine. But heroin can be snorted like cocaine, and a new form of heroin has been available since 1977 which can be used in other ways. This is Persian heroin, which has street names like Persian brown, dava (the Iranian word for medicine), Persian, lemon dope (it requires an acid solution like lemon juice to make it soluble enough for injection), rufus, and Southwest Asian heroin. This Persian heroin can be snorted or smoked, which are the two most common forms of use. It can be smoked by mixing it with conventional tobacco or marijuana. It can also be heated up in powder form and the vapor inhaled through a straw. This method is called "chasing the dragon," something that used to be done only with opium. It can also be eaten. This Persian heroin has created some serious problems, because people who previously ran like hell when opiates like heroin were mentioned are now being seduced into using the drug since they don't have to use needles like "real junkies."

On the street, the common white heroin used by addicts runs about 2 to 6 percent pure. Persian, which is marketed on the street as a dark reddish brown granular powder, tends to run as high as 90 percent pure. The expense of the drug gives it the same snob appeal as cocaine among the more affluent drug users and thus contributes to its reputation as a very hip drug. A tenth of a gram will cost you about $75, while a comparable dose of white heroin will cost about one-third that amount. Some people use it as an "antidote" for coming down from cocaine (particularly if one is freebasing).

Another part of the heroin mystique is generated by addicts' frequent references to the orgasmic rush (initial subjective feelings after taking the drug) brought on by high-quality heroin. The addict quoted above says, "It's like your whole body comes." It is also common to hear people describe the warm feeling that bathes the whole body, creating intense feelings of well-being. This feeling has been compared by many to the sensations surrounding fellatio (oral sex performed on the male). Once addicted, the addict loses interest in actual sex—the drug suffices—unless it's related to getting more heroin (prostitution).

There has been a significant upsurge in heroin abuse among middle-class whites, mainly because people kid themselves into thinking they don't run the same risks as mainlining heroin addicts run. They do! Remember, the Persian heroin is available in much greater purity, and therefore potency. Daily use for about thirty days leads to physical addiction, and withdrawal pains are severe—again, it is strong, high-quality dope. The higher the euphoria, the higher the cost of withdrawal. The same applies to its potential for overdose, which can be life-threatening.

As more and more kids and adults get into trying heroin,

Dangers of Heroin Usage

1. The drug takes over your life. Working, loving, playing, all go down the drain. One becomes totally obsessed with the drug.
2. Physical addiction does not require needle injections of the drug. Smoking Persian heroin can lead to physical and psychological addiction. You can crave the drug and develop a narcotics hunger before you are physically hooked.
3. The death rate associated with 90-percent-pure heroin is much higher than with the low-grade white heroin.
4. Addiction to heroin is damn difficult to shake. Whether it's methadone maintenance or drug-free treatment, the ability to remain heroin-free is a crap shoot at best. You end up either taking methadone for the rest of your life or hoping you are part of the small percentage of people who make it after drug-free treatment.

the peer pressure that used to guarantee that heroin be avoided at all costs is seriously eroding. An article in *High Times* magazine states: "Heroin has become mass hip. Like black leather pants and imported French cigarettes, it confers a special status to its user. With an armful of tracks underneath a Giorgio Armani sports jacket, this year's junkie is no sleazy social leper—he's suddenly fashionable." Treatment programs have been reporting an upsurge in middle-class white addicts since 1977, with no signs of decrease in sight.

Heroin carries a very high benefit/risk ratio with the deck stacked on the side of the risks. The cost of attempting to achieve the special oblivion possible with heroin is the obliteration of your present lifestyle. An addiction to heroin, particularly high-grade heroin, is a nightmare—a nightmare that is happening to nice white middle- and upper-class kids and adults.

SUPER POT

In 1964 two Israeli chemists, Gaoni and Mechoulam, isolated the major psychoactive substance in marijuana, 1-delta-9-trans-tetrahydrocannabinol, more commonly referred to as THC. Research is underway involving other cannabinoids with names like cannabicyclol, cannabichromene, cannabigerol, cannabivarol, and cannabidivarol to learn what role they play in intoxification and related phenomena like the "munchies," the insatiable eating behavior sometimes associated with pot smoking. What is known is that the more THC, the stronger the high. The three main strains of cannabis are *Cannabis sativa,* with its familiar star-shaped leaf, native to North America; *Cannabis indicta,* an import from Asia, more potent than *sativa; Cannabis ruderalis,* an import from the Soviet Union, now being referred to as the latest "super-strain." As a rule *sativa* contains the least THC, *indicta* more, and *ruderalis* the most. Thanks to Yankee ingenuity all three strains have been cultivated as sinsemilla. Sinsemilla is Spanish for "without seeds." Cannabis is remarkable for being able to change its sex. Under certain conditions, male plants can turn into female plants and vice versa. Plants grown from seeds from far-flung corners of the world will take on characteristics of the local strain after three generations. These are hearty and versatile plants. Sinsemilla is marijuana without the male plants. Growers cull out the males the moment their sex characteristics are spotted. Female plants put out more resins and therefore more THC. According to one aficionado, "You get high on sinsemilla and you get stoned on Colombian." Sinsemilla is the pot smoker's plant of choice and sells for $250 to $300 per ounce. A lot of it is grown in California, making certain parts of that state a veritable marijuana farmers' market.

There are other super pot strains around and most of them are imports. They go under such names as Puna Butter, Maui Wowie, Thai Sticks, Panama Red, Acapulco Gold, Kuna Gold, and ganja (Jamaica). The main point is that due to the greatly increased THC content, this super pot should command a great deal of respect and cautionary warnings, particularly for novices. The *sativa* that America grew up on in the 1960s is far less potent than the super pot of the '80s. Even experienced *sativa* users find that the *indica* and sinsemilla plants will get them "very, very stoned" and that the high will last for many hours. Users of super pot, sometimes called "exotic," have reported going to sleep stoned and waking up stoned the next morning. One used to hear stories about many people failing to get high the first few times they smoked. This happened mostly with *sativa* and is far less likely to occur with the newer, more powerful strains. First-time users of the new stuff are getting extremely stoned. Motor coordination, concentration, balance, speech, clear thinking are all profoundly affected. If you have an opportunity to try these forms of marijuana, take one toke, at the most two, and then wait a while. Failure to titrate the dose in this manner can lead to very lengthy and intense drug experiences. Again, moderation and common sense are the hallmarks of judicious drug use. Failure to use them could lead to some very bad trips, even for experienced smokers. Many smokers report a tolerance effect in which once used to the stronger strains they cannot go back to the less potent stuff. While this type of tolerance may not lead to dependence, it can lead you into more expensive purchases than you can handle. Once you are spending money on drugs that should be going for other things like rent and food, you have a drug problem. You can't necessarily trust someone else's "head" to guide your pot experiences. Not only do strains differ in potency, but the placebo effect (realizing drug effects because they are expected) can cause one smoker to differ greatly in the subjective drug experience from any other smoker.

COMBINING DRUGS

A new word has entered into our vocabulary: polypharmacy. It means using more than one drug, sometimes at the same time, sometimes separately.

The use of any drug involves a fine balance between benefits and risks. When you put two drugs together, this equation becomes a lot more complicated and dangerous. While many drug combinations are possible, the one most prevalent in the studies done by treatment people and researchers is alcohol in combination with other drugs. An educated physician (up-to-date on drug interactions) or pharmacist will warn you about the potential hazards of mixing alcohol with certain prescription and over-the-counter (OTC) medications. Who will warn you about combining alcohol with street drugs, or street drugs with licit drugs? You will need to know some terminology to proceed with your education.

Tolerance: As your body adapts to drugs over time, certain tissues react less vigorously to the drug's presence. This cumulative resistance to the pharmacological effects of a drug is called tolerance. It has occurred when the repeated use of a given dose produces a decreased effect. This means that the person will have to take increased doses to get the original effect.

Cross-tolerance: After tolerance to a specific drug has developed, tolerance to others in the same or a related drug class will also be present. Example: someone tolerant to a barbiturate will also be tolerant to other barbiturates, other sedatives, alcohol, and the minor tranquilizers.

Synergism: When two drugs act similarly, they are said to be synergistic.

Antagonism: When two drugs have opposing effects, they are said to be antagonists. An example would be Narcan (naloxone), a narcotic that is antagonistic when combined with heroin.

Additive: When two drugs acting similarly are used together and the result is a simple summation of effect, they are said to be additive. An example is combining Scotch and wine.

Supra-additive: Also called *potentiation.* When the effect of two synergistic drugs is greater than the sum of their doses, they are said to be supra-additive. An example is combining alcohol and sedatives like the barbiturates.

In order to see how the kinds of chemical interactions listed above actually work, let us use one type of mixture: alcohol and another drug. Alcohol (ethanol is what the chemists call it) is a central nervous system (CNS) depressant and a general anesthetic. It has the capacity, like other anesthetics, to cause an initial depression of the inhibitory control mechanism. That's why we feel free and loose when we first drink. However, as more alcohol is added to the human body the CNS gets further depressed and sedated. The chemical interactions listed below occur at a cellular level and are not under conscious control. The only thing you can really control is what and how much goes into your body—after that, involuntary systems take over.

Many people are ignorant about the negative effects of combining drugs; others deliberately combine drugs to get a "better" high. It is known that the majority of drug-dependent persons, some 80 percent, abused alcohol before becoming addicted to other drugs. The literature also reflects the fact that about 30 percent of drug-dependent people use alcohol as a substitute for

Alcohol and Other Drug Combinations

If a person drinks and also uses:	This is what can happen:
Narcotics (heroin, morphine, methadone, etc.)	Effect is additive. Addicts are very vulnerable to liver disease. This combination is a frequent cause of death in addicts. Darvon (propoxyphene) users should exercise great care as this drug closely resembles methadone in its chemical structure.
Sedatives (barbiturates, hypnotics, hypnotic-sedatives)	Effects are supra-additive. Sedatives and alcohol both produce tolerance and cross-tolerance. Both are addicting and the withdrawal syndrome is identical. Combination has a powerful effect on mental and motor tasks: it worsens performance. This can lead to accidental suicide because of supra-additive aspect.
Minor tranquilizers (Valium, Librium, Miltown, Equanil, etc.)	Effects are additive. Combination causes increased sedation and can interfere with both concentration and coordination. In high enough amounts it can be lethal.
Marijuana	The THC (delta-9-tetrahydrocannabinol) in grass has a sedative effect, and combined with alcohol the effects are additive. Cross-tolerance has not been established. Motor skills and coordination worsen with this combo.
Stimulants (amphetamines, Ritalin, caffeine, etc.)	The initial excitability and disinhibition of alcohol can be synergistic with amphetamines, leading to overactivity and in-

240

If a person drinks and also uses:	This is what can happen:
	ducement of increased hostility and paranoia. Blood alcohol levels are unaffected by caffeine, even though some people report feeling more "wide awake." Coffee does not sober anyone up.
Antidepressants (Elavil, Nardil, Marplan, Sinequan, Parnate, Tofranil, Vivactyl, Norpramin, etc.)	Antidepressants are not stimulants. They have a sedative quality. Depending on which antidepressants and what kind of alcoholic beverage, the reactions can include excess sedation, incoordination, stomach upset, dangerously high blood pressure, and death.
Antihistamines (Benadryl, Chlor-Trimeton, etc.)	Effects are additive in terms of sedation. Antihistamines are present in many OTCs, so read the ingredients on the label. Interaction impairs motor and mental coordination.

their preferred drug of abuse, as well as a means of boosting, balancing, counteracting, and sustaining the effects of other drugs. People who use psychotropic (mind-altering) drugs indiscriminately are called "garbage heads" and run a high risk of dangerous interactions. Alcohol abuse and alcoholism are significant problems for former drug abusers who have gone through drug-free rehabilitation programs, as well as those on methadone maintenance programs. In one major study of over 1000 alcoholics in treatment it was found that 44 percent of them used drugs (mainly tranquilizers and barbiturates) before treatment of their alcoholism and 30 percent after treatment. Treatment programs in the fields of both alcoholism and drug abuse report that the multiple (sometimes called polydrug) abuser suffers from more problems than the single-substance abuser. The polydrug patients have more significant medical, psychological, and adjustment problems and have poorer prognoses than the users of one drug. Their histories read like waking nightmares, with a great deal of family pathology in their backgrounds.

Many drugs alter time perception so that you think a lot of time has passed when in fact only minutes have gone by. When drugs are combined, this distortion of time perception is even greater. Better make sure you use a watch or clock to judge time. And remember to titrate the dose(s); otherwise, combining drugs can lead to the hospital emergency room, the psychiatric ward, or even the cemetery!

SEX AND DRUGS

SALLY: Sex is sooooo nice when you drop a lude!

RALPH: Ludes slow me down too much. Have you ever tried poppers [amyl or butyl nitrate] just before orgasm? That will really blow your mind.

SUSAN: Poppers make me dizzy and give me a headache but the orgasm is real nice.

JOE: You're all crazy. The only drug to take when you're having sex is cocaine. You feel so intense that everything seems to explode. Don't waste your time with that other shit!

PHIL: My wife and I prefer some good grass or a little hash oil. We really get into some long and lazy loving when we are high.

JANE: I think you're all very silly and have missed the point. Sex is so much fun, why does anyone need drugs to get off? Okay, once in a while you might want to ball when you are stoned, but only once in a while.

This conversation took place among upper-middle-class adults. No junkies in the group. They all use drugs in a way they consider fun and safe. They are quick to defend their drug(s) of choice and can rhapsodize for hours about the virtues of getting high.

Some people will find these practices amusing; others will find them sad, still others will find them alarming, or interesting, or informative. People have plenty of opinions about the use of drugs and plenty of opinions about human sexuality. When you ask them about both together, you'd better stand back because no one can remain neutral about a topic like this. There are a lot of myths, folklore, old wives' tales, and just plain nonsense surrounding the use of drugs and human sexuality. Pro- and antidrug groups both tend to mislead us about these complicated human behaviors. In their extreme rigidities, each tends to oversimplify and generalize. Somewhere in between lies the truth.

The first step in unraveling the mystery is to have a clear understanding of just what mechanism controls human sexuality. Here is one woman's opinion:

> My sexuality is many different things about me. The way I wear my hair, my clothes, my perfume, the way I speak. I think it may come out more in the attitudes that I project than the way I actually look. The way I come on to people can be very sexual or asexual. The jokes I tell are the easiest way for me to talk about sex. I am aware of my sexual self even when I am not engaged in overt sexual activity. My imagination can fire up my body. I guess the easiest way to say it is that my whole being is involved in my sexuality.

The most powerful sex organ in the human body is the brain! The brain and central nervous system make up the command center for all human functioning, including sex. It's the brain, with its marvelous ability to remember past delights and project future ones, that stands at the center of our sexual lives and functioning.

Sex is used to sell just about every imaginable product. Cosmetics, clothing, alcohol, cars, cigarettes, motorcycles, hair-care products, and on and on. Sex is used to sell drugs too. Many drugs, both licit and illicit, promise enhanced sexuality. Look at all those happy couples sensuously sipping beer, wine, and hard liquor. Check out some of the sex publications and see what products they are advertising—everything from placebo sex aids to vitamin E. Let's take a closer look at the concept of a placebo, because it is central to the sex and drugs issue. A placebo effect is any effect attributed to a drug that is not actually a consequence of the pharmacological properties of the drug. Mental set is what determines that a placebo will work. I once witnessed three out of four people claim to be stoned after smoking what they thought was marijuana. It was actually conventional tobacco and some dried leaves (all four were regular cigarette smokers). Medical research is full of dramatic examples of the placebo effect. If your mental set is that the drug is going to turn you on sexually and the setting is conducive to expressing your sexuality, then your wish will probably come true. People have an amazing ability to fool themselves. We fill our heads with illusions about what drugs will do for our sex lives, and then someone will come along who can profit from that illusion. Voilà—the drug is purchased, and then taken, and . . . Sometimes it works and sometimes it doesn't. Sometimes our heads fool our bodies and sometimes they don't.

Many people are inhibited and uptight when it comes to such things as joyfully acknowledging their sexual selves, exploring their own bodies, sharing fantasies with partners, enjoying sex without guilt, enjoying sex without the fear of not performing well, coming on to someone sexually, and speaking freely about the subject. Part of that inhibition and tension is also the failure to take proper care of our health (body and mind). Obesity, cigarette smoking, flaccid muscles, short wind, and the like all impede sexual enjoyment. In addition, the media has us believing that if we are not constantly aroused sexual athletes we have failed! We buy the hype and end up believing that everyone else is having a better time in bed than we are. So off we go into our sexual adventures carrying a lot of anxiety, guilt, self-doubt, fear of failure, and hope for the best. And then someone says "Hey man, sex is better with drugs! Get with it! Turn on and enjoy!"

People have been searching for the perfect aphrodisiac for thousands of years. Spanish Fly is a ground-up beetle called cantharides, which burns the lining of the bladder and urethra and reflexly stimulates the sexual organs. It causes erection of the clitoris, engorgement of the labia, and tingling of the vagina in women, and causes an immense and painful erection in men. It can also cause ulcers throughout the intestinal tract and dysentery. It can cause convulsions and death. How did this dangerous drug earn its reputation as an aphrodisiac? Because people foolishly interpreted the bladder and urethral irritation as sexual arousal.

According to doctors and scientists there is no true aphrodisiac. It's either the placebo effect or a misinterpretation like the one about Spanish Fly. If the drug we take is defined as an aphrodisiac and we expect it to cause sexual arousal, then the odds are that it will.

The word "aphrodisiac" comes from the name of the Greek goddess of love, Aphrodite. It applies to something that increases sexual desire or excitement. Scientists may insist on well-controlled double-blind studies of aphrodisiacs before calling them by that name, but there is no doubt that drugs do indeed affect sexual desire and excitement.

A wide variety of drugs enhance or interfere with sexual functioning. As for pharmaceuticals you can obtain from your doctor, you will probably discover that the doctor is just as uptight when it comes to talking about sex as you are. However, since some drugs are real sexual downers, it is important that you overcome your timidity and ask if any of the prescribed drugs or OTCs you are taking can adversely affect your sex life. (Do not start or stop taking a drug without first discussing it with your doctor.)

How any drug will affect you sexually depends on how much you take. Shakespeare said it best when it comes to drinking too much alcohol:

. . . it provokes the desire, but it takes away from the performance . . .

Macbeth

In the drug scene this is known as going "one toke over the line." When people get high they often feel amorous, but too

Drugs That May Interfere with Sexual Functioning[4]

alcohol (in large enough amounts or used chronically)

alseroxylon (Rau-Tab, Rautensin, Rauwiloid)

amphetamines (high dose or chronic use)

anabolic steroids

atropine (antispasmodic elixir)

barbiturates

belladonna

bethadidine

butaperazine (Repoise)

chlordiazepoxide (Librium)

chlorpromazine (Thorazine)

chlorprothixene (Taractan)

chlorthalidone (Hygroton)

cimetidine (Tagamet)

clofibrate (Atromid-S)

clonidine (Catapres)

cyproterone acetate

debrisoquine

deserpidine (Harmonyl)

desipramine (Norpramin, Pertofrane)

diazepam (Valium)

dicyclomine (Bentyl)

diethylpropion (Tenuate)

diethylstilbestrol (Stilphostrol, Tylosterone)

disopyramide (Norpace)

disulfiram (Antabuse)

doxepin (Adapin, Sinequan)

estrogens

fenfluramine (Pondimin)

fluphenazine (Prolixin)

furosemide (Lasix)

guanethidine (Esimil, Ismelin)

haloperidol (Haldol)

heroin

hydralazine (Apresoline, Lopress)

hydromorphone (Dilaudid)

imipramine (Tofranil)

isocarboxazid (Marplan)

levodopa (Bendopa, Dopar, Levopa)

lithium (Eskalith, Lithane, Lithonate)

mazindol (Sanorex)

mebanazine (Actomol)

meperidine (Demerol)

mesoridazine (Serentil)

methadone

methantheline (Banthine)

methscopolamine (Pamine)

methyldopa (Aldomet, Aldoclor, Aldoril)

morphine

nicotine

nortriptyline (Aventyl, Pamelor)

opium

oral contraceptives

pargyline (Eutonyl)

perphenazine (Trilafon)

phenelzine (Nardil)

phenmetrazine (Preludin)

phenoxybenzamine (Dibenzyline)

prazosin (Minipress)

prochlorperazine (Compazine)

propantheline (Probanthine)	thioridazine (Mellaril)
protriptyline (Vivactyl)	thiothixene (Navane)
rauwolfia (Raudixin,	tranylcypromine (Parnate)
Raupena, Rauserpa)	triamterene (Dyrenium)
rescinnamine (Moderil)	trifluoperazine (Stelazine)
reserpine (Serpasil, Diupres)	tryptophan
scopolamine	
thiazide diuretics (Hydrodi-	
uril)	

much of any drug can mess you up either physically or mentally and make sex less than enjoyable or even impossible.

Alcohol and other drugs alter perception, change moods, block out certain stimuli from within and without, dissolve inhibitions against many things including sex, reduce anxiety, and the like. They do this by intervening in various biochemical processes in the body (many of which are in the central nervous system—

Drugs That May Enhance or Increase Sexuality[4]

alcohol (in small amounts, varies from person to person)	hashish/hash oil
	isobutyl nitrite
	LSD (d-lysergic acid diethylamide tartrate 25)
amphetamines (in small amounts)	marijuana
amyl nitrite	MDA (methylenedioxyamphetamine)
androgens (Methyltestosterone)	mescaline
barbiturates (in small amounts, very similar to alcohol)	methaqualone (Sopor, Parest, Quaalude), (in small amounts)
bromocriptine (Parlodel)	peyote
butyl nitrite	psilocybin
cocaine	STP (2,5-Dimethoxy-4-methylamphetamine) (DOM)
DMT (dimethyltryptamine)	
glutethimide (Doriden)	

the command center). The body undergoes a chemical change brought about by the drug. On a behavioral level we interpret these changes based on expectations, set, and setting. Our drug-taking can influence actual sex at any one of the four phases of the sexual response in men and women.

Excitement: Different things turn on different people, leading to erection, lubrication—initial arousal.

Plateau: Body completes readiness for sexual activity: full erection of penis and clitoris, more lubrication, nipples become erect.

Orgasm: Peak of activity leading to ejaculation and orgasm. Stimulation leads to pleasure and involuntary muscle contractions in both men and women.

Resolution: Rest period after orgasm. Women if aroused again do not require a rest; men, on the other hand, seem to require rest before continuing.

All kinds of claims are made for the drugs that enhance sex. It appears that most impact on the excitement phase. By disinhibiting many of the psychological and emotional blocks to arousal, drugs allow people to "turn on" sexually after turning on with drugs. All those fears and hang-ups about technique, should-I-shouldn't-I, and morality often dissolve in the admixture of natural desires and mind-altering drugs. Since getting high violates social custom and having sex often does the same, it is no wonder that the two activities seem to go hand in hand.

Some people use drugs because they want to block out all thoughts and ideas and experience only feelings. It is probably true that those who indulge in casual sex need drugs like ludes or alcohol to attain an "I just want to ball" attitude. Uncomfortable with the "meat rack" approach to human relations, they have to get stoned first. Many pornographic films portray the seduction of reluctant women by means of marijuana, alcohol, and other drugs. The idea is that social inhibition is the only barrier to unfettered sexuality and that women need to be "set free" by men. It's time we laid this ancient stereotype to rest.

Some people use drugs to slow down the sexual response so that they may savor it longer. This often applies to foreplay and afterplay—or to actual intercourse. Afterplay is one of the most neglected aspects of sexuality. Real time may not change, but in a stoned condition people may feel as if they are spending more time in sex play. Sometimes real time is prolonged, as with the topical application of cocaine to the sexual organs.

Others may use drugs to gain a sense of potency and sexual energy or to intensify orgasm. The inhalants, which go under many different names (Aroma of Man, Locker Room, Oz, Rush, Bolt, Heart On, Hi Baller, to name just a few), are available without prescription. These volatile inhalants are actually amyl nitrite, butyl nitrite, and isobutyl nitrite. Only amyl nitrite requires a prescription. Commonly called poppers or snappers because you have to break the ampule (hence the popping sound), these drugs are said to give a powerful lift to orgasm if sniffed just before you reach that state. This will require you to stop what you are doing to break the ampule and inhale the drug. While users report various pleasurable effects, the drugs do have a rather pungent odor and can cause dizziness and headaches. Kids like to sniff this stuff to get high even if they are not having sex.

Some people in the drug scene use sex as a commodity. Most of us are familiar with the stories about women heroin addicts who sell their bodies to support their habits. Heroin inhibits the achievement of orgasm and ejaculation in men but does not inhibit the ability to achieve and maintain an erection. A particularly handsome fellow whose current girlfriend was a former beauty queen had an interesting quid pro quo going. He kept her in lengthy love-making sessions and she kept him in drugs.

Many drug-using people remain convinced that the drugs are creating and not merely enhancing their sexuality. Actually, all the drugs are really doing is releasing something that already exists within us. Drugs create a temporary illusion during which we are no longer alienated from our bodies, where guilt, sin, and shame dissolve, and where we are freed from the "tyranny of the orgasm." It is easier to stop worrying about technique and the mechanics of sexuality when you are stoned.

Perhaps more than anything else, the drugs help people to relax. When we are relaxed we are much freer to enjoy sex. It seems that millions of Americans have a problem being able to relax enough to really enjoy sex. Sexuality is a combination of the mind, the body, and the spirit all bound up in the joyful act of giving and receiving. Drugs can become unnecessary for many when they find nonchemical ways to freer sexual expression.

SEX AND DRUGS QUESTIONNAIRE

True   False

1. Do you and your partner(s) often get high before making love?
2. Is sex better when you use drugs than when you don't?
3. Do you, when planning a night of love-making, make sure that you have a supply of drugs (including alcohol)?
4. When combining sex and drugs, do you ever have trouble remembering what happened the night before?
5. Do you have trouble relaxing sexually without drugs?
6. Have drugs ever messed up your sexual performance?
7. Do you stop in the middle of lovemaking to get high?
8. Do you use drugs to "seduce" your partner(s)?

GETTING HIGH

True   False

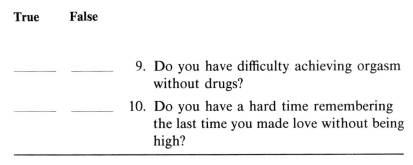

_____   _____   9. Do you have difficulty achieving orgasm without drugs?

_____   _____   10. Do you have a hard time remembering the last time you made love without being high?

Scoring key: 1–3 "true": Drugs are playing a role in your sex life. Is that what you really want?

4–6 "true": You have come to rely quite heavily on drugs to ensure feeling states that can be achieved without them.

7–10 "true": Your sex life is totally dependent upon the use of drugs. You have a problem with drugs that requires treatment. Better check out your sexual functioning after you are drug-free for a while to see if you have a problem in that area as well.

Everything exists in contrast to something else. Sex and drugs are nicer when sex without drugs is good. If you can get it on only with drugs, then something is wrong. Ninety percent of sex therapy is psychotherapy; it is often our emotional selves that need sorting out in order to find sexual fulfillment. Drugs can achieve this, but it is strictly short-term. Why? Because it's "state-dependent" sexuality; you'll have to get high to get back to that "state" each time. You can end up with a functional addiction—believing that good sex without the drugs is impossible. It is better to get there without the drugs and then perhaps choose to use them once in a while for variety. I have treated many drug-related sexual burnouts. In most cases there is nothing physically wrong. The problems are more in the areas of body image, guilt, clumsiness, and fear of rejection. These people ended up trading their lovers for a drug habit. It happens without their realizing what is happening.

It happens in adolescence in two distinctly polarized ways. One way is for kids to get into the drug scene to the exclusion of all else—thereby successfully avoiding (at least for the moment)

251

any confrontation with their own sexuality. Then there are the "lovers," who get into drugs and sex but who really exchange nothing of emotional value with their partners.

Sex and Drugs

- Your date may not want or need any drugs to be interested in sex. Some folks get insulted if they think you need to get high to enjoy their company.
- Titrate the dose.
- Remember, it's your brains that are in charge—so be careful how you feed your head.
- Everybody is different in how they enjoy sex. Stay loose and be open.
- Getting stoned is a good way to end up pregnant. Take care of business in the birth control department before getting high.
- If you need drugs to enjoy sex, it's time to seek some professional help.
- Drugs or no drugs, don't say yes when you want to say no.
- Sex talk and shared fantasies are a great turn-on.
- Good sex is not the exclusive playground of the young and the beautiful.
- Don't get hung up with technique. Let it flow and enjoy the giving and receiving of pleasure. Guide your lover. Tell him or her what you like.
- Variety is the spice of life. Make love at different hours, in new places. Surprise each other. Try different things.
- It's very helpful to realize that if you take care of your body, your body will take care of you. Keep in shape and stay healthy.

ETIQUETTE

Like few other images, the character of the pusher stirs up deep-seated emotions. There is a special kind of revulsion for the person who sells drugs. Many people say, "If we just clean up the pushers, everything will be all right!" Aside from the fact that consumer demand is what so dramatically affects supplies, our definition of pusher has been too narrow. Many people "push" drugs, if we define the term to mean the sale, promotion, and use of mind-altering substances. Besides the street drug dealer, the list includes doctors, pharmacists, patients, liquor stores, grocery stores selling beer, advertising agencies, sellers and manufacturers of prescription and OTC drugs—and family members, friends, cultural gurus, trend setters, and party hosts and hostesses. Modern-day party throwers can and do supply their guests with the widest assortment of drinkables, smokables, popables, snortables, and eatables (food is a mood changer and reinforcer). Where once an adequately supplied bar would suffice, many party givers now feel compelled to offer good grass or cocaine.

Social competition is fast and furious in some sets, and finding a good connection (pusher) isn't all that easy. Some catering houses now ask if the revelers will require a "smoking room" set aside from the general festivities.

Bars in the home have become a status symbol among the middle class. According to the *Summary of the 3rd Annual Report on Alcohol and Health* submitted to the U.S. Congress by the Secretary of Health, Education and Welfare (1978):

> The nation's per capita consumption of alcoholic beverages increased during the 1960s, in a trend generally attributed to more liberal alcohol control laws, to an increased proportion of young people in the population, and to a higher number of women drinking. Per capita consumption, based on sales data, has risen little since 1971, ranging from 2.63 to 2.69 gallons of absolute ethanol (ethyl alcohol) per person 14 years of age and older. This consumption level is the highest recorded since 1850.

As a host or hostess you must use some wisdom in your role as "drug pusher" at your parties. You will provide the chemicals, the setting in which they will be used, and you may in fact set the tone for the use of these chemicals. You are not responsible for what your guests do—that is their own affair—but you must accept responsibility for the setting, and you should be prepared to aid your guests if they get into trouble. Attention to these matters can mean the difference between a good time and a disaster.

A new variable is creeping into the selection process when guest lists for parties are drawn up: knowing who does and does not use a variety of drugs. If getting high is a central theme of the party, then you would not want to put nonusers in the embarrassing position of feeling like oddballs. They may become hostile and defensive, say things like "I don't need that to have a good time," and make an early exit. If drugs define part of the good time at your party, then some thoughtfulness about heterogeneous and homogeneous crowds is in order.

Another thing to keep in mind is the physical setting. Most of us don't enjoy crowded quarters; crowding breeds aggression. Many people when faced with crowds drift into other parts of the house where you may not want them to go. So attention to space is important. If you don't want people openly using drugs like grass or cocaine, you should provide a room for this separate purpose—otherwise you may notice some funny odors emanating from the bathroom. If, on the other hand, you don't wish people to do this in your home, do not assume they know that. A discreet comment away from the hearing of others is in order. Don't be surprised if they get high anyway.

Having a bartender who can exercise some discretion is a good idea. Volunteers often turn out to be unintentional pushers, pouring with a heavy hand. It's a good idea to make use of a shot glass rather than guesstimates of how much one is pouring. It is not necessary to pour doubles, either. People can always come back for more. Don't feel compelled to constantly foist drinks or other chemicals on your guests. Wait until drink glasses are empty, and check out your guests' behavior. If someone says "No thanks," don't feel that you must keep offering. If you are providing other drugs, then reasonable amounts are indicated, especially if you are providing high-grade stuff.

One of the more difficult things you may be called upon to deal with is setting limits for your guests. When someone has had too much drink, drug, or food (overeating or eating chemically altered foods), you should directly express your concern for them. How much is too much? This is tricky, but things like being overly boisterous, stuporous, hostile, or intimidating, being sick to one's stomach, slurring speech, bumping into things, spilling food or drinks all qualify as danger signs. Your own common sense and your expectation that people should respect your property and other guests is a good rule of thumb. You are not obligated, in any sense of the term, to provide another drink or toke or whatever to a guest who can't handle it. It's better to risk their ire on the spot, followed by a sober conversation the next day. If they can't "forgive" you, it's their problem, not yours. If they are experiencing a real problem with drugs, then at least you did not add to it.

It's a good idea to serve nonalcoholic drinks in addition to the beer, wine, and liquor. Some people don't drink alcohol. Those getting high on other chemicals may not wish to combine them with alcohol (generally a wise thing not to do). Serving snacks will slow down the rate at which alcohol is absorbed into the bloodstream. If people pig down a lot of drugs and booze and end up stoned out of their minds, you may begin to wonder just what the original intent of the party was anyway. You will be right to be concerned if the chemicals seem to be the sole source of fun at your party.

If you are into herbal cooking (as in marijuana, hashish, mescaline, psilocybin) or esoterica from the bar, give your guests fair warning about the special ingredients. As a rule, drugs that are eaten take longer to be absorbed through the stomach lining (as compared with the lungs or nasal mucosa), and there is a "delayed" reaction. However, when the high registers it tends to be strong and last quite a while. So don't get carried away with psychoactive ingredients. If using potent potables like overproof rum (151 proof) or strong tequila (the one with the fermentation worms at the bottom), be sure to tell your guests to expect an extra jolt, and to watch how many drinks they consume.

For those of you who have planned a whole evening of food and drink, let your guests know so that they can plan their drug use accordingly. Cannabis products (marijuana, hashish, hash oil) with a lot of 9-delta-THC (researchers think this is what causes "the munchies") have a tendency to cause overeating. Cocaine is a powerful appetite suppressant, so it's best served after dinner. (Some diet clinics do a heavy underground business in cocaine and amphetamines.)

If you are serving different alcoholic beverages before, during, and after the meal, let your guests know this so they can choose between your yummy cooking and their mood changers. Many hosts and hostesses have learned the hard way to bring out the nonalcoholic chemicals after the meal.

Be very careful with leftovers of herbal cooking. Some Alice B. Toklas brownies (brownies cooked with marijuana or hashish) stashed in a friend's refrigerator were discovered by the babysitter. This fifteen-year-old girl ate a whole brownie and then started to feel very weird. Her mother had to take over the babysitting chores while she went home and fell asleep. This created a moral dilemma for the owner of the brownies, who ultimately decided to tell the sitter's parents the truth. The girl was fine and the parents took it in stride, but sometimes things do not work out so well.

John's story

John did not know the punch had been spiked with LSD. He ate a lot of pretzels and potato chips and drank a lot of punch to deal with his thirst. When he began tripping it seemed pleasant at first. Then things got very scary. John felt like he was going crazy. His father came to the party and drove John to the nearest emergency room. No one told either John or his father about the acid. John was admitted to the psychiatric unit suffering from what appeared to be paranoid schizophrenia, the worst of all the mental illnesses. It took two days on the unit plus the knowledge that John had ingested LSD (thanks to an anonymous phone call) for everything to return to normal.

DRINKING, DRUGGING, AND DRIVING: A PRESCRIPTION FOR DEATH

On average, alcohol is metabolized by the human body at the rate of one ounce per hour. That's the equivalent of one shot glass of distilled spirits, one can of beer, or one glass of wine. This amount of alcohol will yield a .02 percent level of blood alcohol content (BAC). The chart listed below will help you to determine your blood alcohol content based on your body weight and the number of drinks you have consumed over a given period of time. This chart is based upon New York State law where over .05 percent BAC is considered driving while impaired and .10 percent and up is considered driving while intoxicated (DWI).

Body Weight	DRINKS (Two hour period)											
100	1	2	3	4	5	6	7	8	9	10	11	12
120	1	2	3	4	5	6	7	8	9	10	11	12
140	1	2	3	4	5	6	7	8	9	10	11	12
160	1	2	3	4	5	6	7	8	9	10	11	12
180	1	2	3	4	5	6	7	8	9	10	11	12
200	1	2	3	4	5	6	7	8	9	10	11	12
220	1	2	3	4	5	6	7	8	9	10	11	12
240	1	2	3	4	5	6	7	8	9	10	11	12

BAC= Blood Alcohol Content	Caution. . . Keep your BAC under .04%	Driving While Impaired above .05%	Driving While Intoxicated (DWI) .10% and up
	You're playing it safe	First offense • $250 fine • up to 15 days in jail • 90-day loss of license	First conviction: • $350–500 fine • Up to one year in jail • Possible three-year probation • Minimum six-months loss of license

Most states use the .10 percent to determine the DWI standard. Check your own state laws.

No amount of coffee, cold showers, fresh air, or food will increase the rate of metabolism. What coffee and food will do is give the person more nondrinking time and allow for the alcohol already in the system to be metabolized (broken down chemically and excreted through urine or sweating). All you get when you give coffee to someone who has had too much to drink is a wide-awake drunk! The Food and Drug Administration (FDA) has issued a warning against products that purportedly sober people up, stating that there is no scientific proof that anything can minimize inebriation and stressing that no drug has been approved for that purpose. "The FDA is unaware of adequate and well-controlled scientific studies which demonstrate that any product or ingredient can prevent or minimize inebriation. There is an obvious danger if motorists, in particular, rely on a product's claims that it will sober them up unless such claims are substantiated."

A common problem at parties is the person who has had too much to drink or drug. The central issue becomes what to do after you have shared your polite concern, you have closed the bar, you have stopped passing out other drugs, and someone is in trouble. You have already taken the first important step by seeing to it that this person does not put any more drugs into his or her system. Your second concern must be to see that he or she gets home safely. If this is impossible, be prepared to let the person sleep it off at your place. Under no circumstances should you allow this person to drive a car! Let me share some awesome statistics with you in the hope that none of your guests will ever be counted among these chilling numbers.

- Drunk drivers kill 25,000 men, women, children, and babies each year on American highways. They injure another 750,000. That is nearly 70 persons killed and 2,054 seriously injured each and every day.
- In New York State, between one-third and one-half of all fatal accidents involve a driver who has been drinking.

258

Over 1,000 persons were killed by drunk drivers in 1980; another 20,000 persons were seriously injured.

- Drunk driving is the leading killer of our youth, those age fifteen to twenty-four, in New York. Motor vehicle accidents harm more than three times as many New Yorkers as do cancer, heart disease, and stroke combined.

- Added to this horrifying human toll is the economic cost of alcohol-involved car crashes—a total of $702 million in 1979 alone resulting from:

$562 million in lost work or productivity
$4.3 million in increased insurance costs
$60 million in medical costs
$9.7 million in legal and court costs
$54 million in vehicle and property damage
$12 million in a combination of funeral costs, accident investigations, and traffic delays.

In a study conducted by the Eagleton Institute of Politics at Rutgers University in 1982, it was found that one in four New Jersey drivers (27 percent) admitted to drinking alcoholic beverages while driving. Of those who were between eighteen and twenty-nine years old, 43 percent said they drank while driving, and 38 percent of all the men questioned admitted doing so. In addition, two-thirds of the men thirty and older and half of all the men interviewed (a total of 503) said they had been at the wheel when passengers were drinking.

Grass-roots activity has begun a ground swell of popular support for tougher drunk driving laws. Spearheaded by a California-based organization known as Mothers Against Drunk Drivers (MADD), the outcry for changes in the law is getting results. In April of 1982 President Reagan created a special commission to combat drunken driving. "Americans are outraged that such slaughter can take place on our highways. The mood of the nation is ripe to make headway to solving the problem," the President said. The commission's first recommendation urges all states to raise the drinking age to twenty-one, as Maryland and New Jersey did recently. Congress has approved grants to states that tighten their drunk driving laws as has been done in New York and seventeen other states. For example, as indicated in the blood alcohol level chart, a drunk driver (DWI) in New York State pays a minimum fine of $350 and loses his or her license for six months. For information on how to contact MADD and similar organizations consult Appendix C: Where to Find Help. Legal limits have not been established for drugs other than alcohol, and there are no incidence and prevalence statistics for the relationship between them and highway accidents and fatalities. This is an area that requires more research. Alcohol in combination with other drugs probably accounts for a significant number of vehicular problems.

Back to our stoned party guest. If he or she came with someone and can get a ride home, that's fine. But if the intoxicated person insists on driving, you must find a way to prevent this. Offer to drive the person home, or have someone else do it. Offer to let him stay over at your home. Stay with him, give him something to eat and some coffee or tea, and don't let him drive until he has sobered up or gotten straight, in the case of drugs. If a person persists in wanting to drive, you can:

1. Take away the car keys and pretend that they are lost.
2. Ask others to help you convince him that it is not safe for him to drive (don't put him down, just state your concern for his safety).
3. Get others to help you if he gets physical. Use restraint only if really necessary.
4. Speak calmly and rationally. People who are loaded are quick to think they are being challenged.

There are things you can do to protect yourself and others from drunk drivers. Wear seat belts and shoulder straps at all times, and ask your passengers to buckle up. Restraints could cut highway casualties in half. Minimize nighttime driving, particularly on weekends. About 80 percent of drunk driving occurs between the hours of 8 P.M. and 8 A.M. Report any suspicious or erratic driving to police.

DEALING WITH ADVERSE DRUG REACTIONS

Denial that anything can happen to us or our friends is responsible for more deaths in the drug scene than anyone cares to acknowledge. The attitude "it can't happen to me" can be a real killer. We tend to see the dangers associated with drugs as happening only to that skid-row wino or that strung-out junkie nodding on the street corner. There are many things that can go wrong in a single administration of a drug. One need not be a junkie to get into trouble. A college student chugalugs a fifth of gin and dies on the spot. Another college student chokes to death on his own vomit after doing a combination of opium and barbiturates. A famous entertainer's daughter walks out of a window on LSD because she thinks she can fly. What about Natalie Wood and William Holden? And Janis Joplin, Jimi Hendrix, John Belushi, Marilyn Monroe, Elvis Presley, and many, many others? Richard Pryor is reported to have almost burned to death while freebasing cocaine. Many of these tragedies could have been prevented.

At large gatherings like rock concerts, there are usually trained medical staff and volunteers to help people who drink or drug too much. It isn't unusual to hear the doctor ask the person who brought the comatose kid into the emergency area, "What did he take?" Too often the answer is, "A red one, a blue one, and a green one." Specific information is needed to treat drug overdoses. When seeking help for someone, you must try to establish what he or she took, how much, and when. This type of information can save lives. Thorazine (chlorpromazine) is a major tranquilizer that is often used to ease the panic reaction which can be part of a "bad trip" on LSD. However, if the person took a different hallucinogenic drug like STP (2,5-dimethoxy-4-methylamphetamine), the use of Thorazine could spell grim news:

Thorazine may potentiate the effects of the STP, which often contains belladonnalike adulterants. Mixing a hallucinogenic drug like DMT (dimethyltryptamine) with chlorpromazine could result in death. Most emergency rooms are using Valium (diazepam) to deal with panic attacks. The adulterants in street drugs and the volatile combinations of multiple drug use make it terribly important that you have factual information. Do not attempt to administer any drugs on your own. Call a doctor or poison control center to find out what to do. If you are stoned your time sense will probably be altered, so use a clock or watch to establish the passage of time. In a party situation it's usually a good idea for the host and/or hostess not to get too loaded. By staying fairly straight you can act as a "shepherd" over your flock. If you find that you have to call for medical assistance, find out what prescription or OTC drugs the person in trouble may have taken, in addition to drugs consumed while partying.

Drinking and drugging can cause or aggravate life-threatening circumstances. Examples are choking, inability to breathe, stroke, and cardiac arrest. If you know basic life support you can save a life. The ABCs of cardiopulmonary resuscitation (CPR) are:

- opening and maintaining an airway (A);
- providing ventilation through rescue breathing (B);
- providing artificial circulation (C) through the use of external cardiac compression.

Basic life support is a two-part emergency first aid procedure. First recognizing the problems: obstructed airway, arrested breathing, and cardiac arrest; and second, properly applying CPR until a victim recovers sufficiently to be transported or until advanced life support is available. Advanced life support is basic life support plus the use of specialized equipment to monitor and drugs to stabilize the patient. Advanced life support is done only by specially trained emergency medical personnel. Courses on CPR are available to all interested persons; you can get more information by contacting the American Heart Association, your family physician, or the cardiology department of your local hospital.

It is estimated that over 650,000 people die from heart attacks every year, with about 350,000 of these deaths occurring outside a hospital, most commonly within two hours after the onset of symptoms. Many other victims die from stroke, automobile accidents, drowning, electrocution, suffocation, and drug intoxification. The more people who know CPR, the more lives can be saved. Listed below are some of the things to look for that might require the application of CPR. These are general guidelines and are not meant as a substitute for taking the formal course.

Warning signs of a heart attack:

1. Pain or discomfort, usually pressure and a burning sensation in the lower chest or upper abdomen. May be a squeezing in the center of the chest which can be severe. People often report that it feels like someone is standing on their chest.
2. These sensations may come and go. The pain can also be felt in the back or shoulder and may spread or radiate into the arms (most often the left arm) or into the jaw or upper abdomen.
3. This type of pain lasting two minutes or more can indicate that a person is having a heart attack.
4. Other symptoms may include sweating, nausea, palpitations (awareness of a fluttering or irregular heartbeat), and shortness of breath.
5. The victim may be pale, or feel faint or dizzy with a sense of impending disaster.

The early warning signs of a heart attack are sometimes confused with indigestion (a risk at all parties). Most people will deny that they are having a heart attack, writing the symptoms off to indigestion, anxiety, or even a passing reaction to drugs taken at the party. The delay in seeking medical attention brought about by this denial can cause the loss of life. It is far better to have the medical experts rule out a coronary event than to let a lay person make this fatal misjudgment.

Warning signs of a stroke:

1. The primary sign is a feeling of sudden, temporary weakness or numbness of the face, arm, and/or leg on one side of the body.
2. Other symptoms include temporary dimness or loss of sight, especially in one eye, and unexplained dizziness, loss of balance, and falls.

When a victim is unconscious, you cannot get him to respond to normal noise, touch, feeling, or pain. This can result from the victim's airway being obstructed, his breathing actually being arrested, or his heart having arrested. Timing is critical: the sooner you reach the victim and determine what procedure to apply, the greater the likelihood of saving a life. It takes only six to ten minutes after the heart stops for permanent brain damage to occur. You must ascertain which of the possible life-threatening conditions prevails. Again, in order to properly learn these steps, you should enroll in a CPR course, where you can learn and practice what to do in an emergency.

Information on assisting a person who is choking is outlined on the following pages.

Some drugs can induce seizures (also referred to as convulsions), particularly in people who are habituated to alcohol and other sedative drugs.

Warning signs of seizures

1. Neck movements, facial twitching, and eyelid blinking.
2. These may progress to include movements of the upper extremities, shoulder, and chest and may also affect the lower extremities. These movements tend to be brief and explosive.
3. Person may make explosive involuntary utterances which can include repetitive obscenities.

When faced with a person having seizures, there are only a limited number of things to do. In the majority of cases the

Choking on food is the sixth leading cause of accidental death—killing more Americans than airplane crashes or firearms. Older people are the most frequent victims of choking, but it can happen to anyone.

Choking most often occurs when
- meat is not cut into small enough pieces
- someone is laughing or talking while chewing
- reflexes are dulled by alcohol
- children are running or playing with food or foreign objects in their mouths

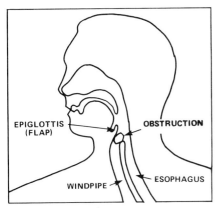

How to recognize choking

Persons who are choking
- suddenly cannot speak, breathe or cough
- may frantically toss their heads or run from the room in panic
- turn blue and finally collapse

SINCE DEATH FROM CHOKING CAN OCCUR WITHIN MINUTES, *SPEED IN REMOVING THE OBJECT WHICH IS BLOCKING THE WINDPIPE IS CRUCIAL.*

First aid for choking

Stand by but **DO NOT INTERFERE WITH A PERSON WHO CAN SPEAK, COUGH OR BREATHE.** If the victim cannot speak, cough or breathe, immediately have someone call for emergency medical help while you take the following action:

FOR A CONSCIOUS VICTIM STANDING OR SITTING

①   **4 back blows**

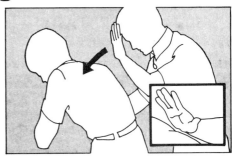

- Stand just behind and to the side of the victim. If necessary, provide support by placing one of your hands on the victim's breast bone. The victim's head should be lower than the victim's chest.
- With the heel of your other hand, give 4 quick, sharp blows between the shoulder blades. If unsuccessful, try...

②   **4 abdominal thrusts**

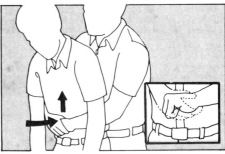

- Stand behind the victim and wrap your arms around his or her waist. Allow the victim's head and upper body to hang forward.
- Make a fist with one hand. Grasp the fist with your other hand, placing the thumb side of the clenched fist against the victim's abdomen— slightly above the navel and below the rib cage.

CAUTION: Make certain your fist is below the rib cage or you may injure the victim!

- With a quick inward and upward thrust, press your fist into the victim's abdomen. Repeat this action 4 times if necessary. (The abdominal thrust is often called "the Heimlich Maneuver" because it was originated by Dr. Henry J. Heimlich, a Cincinnati surgeon.)

REPEAT 4 BACK BLOWS AND 4 QUICK THRUSTS UNTIL THE VICTIM IS NO LONGER CHOKING OR BECOMES UNCONSCIOUS.

FOR A VICTIM LYING DOWN OR UNCONSCIOUS

NOTE: Persons trained in mouth-to-mouth resuscitation may attempt to ventilate an unconscious victim. If ventilation is not immediately successful, begin the following sequence:

 ## 4 back blows

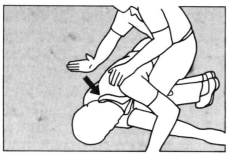

- Roll the victim onto his or her side, facing you, with the victim's chest against your knee.
- With the heel of your hand, give 4 quick, sharp blows between the shoulder blades. If unsuccessful, try...

 ## 4 abdominal thrusts

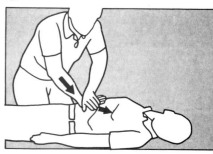

- Roll the victim onto his or her back and take position alongside the victim's hips.
- Place one of your hands on top of the other, with the heel of the bottom hand on the victim's abdomen between the navel and the rib cage. Push in and upward 4 times. Your shoulders should be directly over the victim's abdomen.

 ## clear mouth

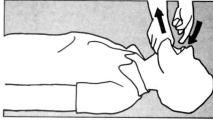

- Check to see if food or object has been dislodged into mouth. Open the victim's mouth by grasping both the tongue and lower jaw between the thumb and fingers and then gently lift the jaw upward.
- Insert the index finger of the other hand down along the inside of the cheek and into the throat as far as the base of the tongue.
- Then use a hooking action to dislodge and remove the food or foreign body. Be careful not to push food back into windpipe.

REPEAT EACH STEP OF THE SEQUENCE UNTIL SUCCESSFUL, STOPPING AS SOON AS THE VICTIM BEGINS BREATHING.

CHOKING FIRST AID FOR INFANTS AND CHILDREN

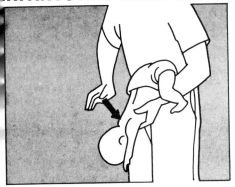

- Place the victim face down on your forearm so that the head is lower than the body.
- Deliver several sharp blows with the heel of your hand to the child's back between the shoulder blades.

SELF HELP
- If you're alone, make a fist with one hand and place thumb side against your abdomen. With the other hand, grasp your fist and press your fist in and upward in sharp, thrusting moves.
- Another method is to press your abdomen forcefully against the back of a chair or a railing, so air is forced out of your lungs to expel the object.

OBTAIN IMMEDIATE MEDICAL CARE

- All choking victims should seek medical care— even if they seem fully recovered. While complications can result from the use of abdominal thrusts on a pregnant woman or someone with a pre-existing medical disorder, first aid for choking should still be used if the victim is in danger of death by choking.

A UNIVERSAL SIGN

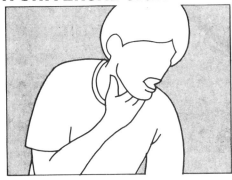

- Efforts have been started to teach a universal sign to use if choking. Signal for help by grasping the neck between the thumb and index finger of one hand.

Source: State of New York, Office of Health Promotion, Department of Health

attacks terminate harmlessly by themselves, regardless of what you do or don't do. People accustomed to dealing with seizures make little of them and do not become excited—this is important for you to keep in mind. *Do not panic!* What you can do is:

- Keep the shirt or blouse collar loose.
- Keep the person away from furniture and other objects which can cause injury.
- If you can, before the teeth are clenched, try to put a soft item between the teeth. Do *not* put your finger in the person's mouth.

Do not make a big fuss when the seizures have passed. Let the victim regain his composure in a separate room and give him something to drink (no alcohol). If this is his first seizure, or if he seems very upset, or if seizures repeat, get him to a hospital or call his doctor. If the recovering victim is too out of it for you to get any relevant information, then medical intervention is in order.

In an Emergency

- Have emergency phone numbers where you can read them quickly.
- Don't panic. Stay calm and think things out carefully.
- Don't hesitate to ask for help from others.
- Don't let denial ("It can't happen to me") stop you from being prepared to deal with an emergency.
- Learn what to do for a choking victim.
- Seriously consider taking a course in CPR.
- Remember the importance of accurate and reliable information about drugs taken (all kinds of drugs).
- Don't try to be a doctor—be an informed and responsive lay person.

Dealing with a bad trip: As a final consideration, let's take a serious look at the psychologically untoward drug reaction. Holistic medicine does not separate the mind, the body, and the spirit. Psychological states influence the body and vice versa. Keep this in mind when dealing with someone who is "freaking out" on drugs.

Anxiety and "blues and blahs" are part of our modern age. The difference between these states of feeling and a reaction to drugs is the intensity of the experience and/or the fact that the victim's condition may be quite upsetting to those nearby. Freaking out or having a bad psychological reaction to a drug (often called a bad trip) has many features:

- severe fright or panic
- extreme anxiety (specific or diffuse)
- profound feelings of sadness
- very distorted body image
- confusion and disorientation
- paranoid ideation
- hallucinations (visual, auditory, or tactile)
- seriously impaired judgment or reasoning ability
- depersonalization
- extreme distractibility
- fear of death
- fear of losing one's mind

The main thing to keep in mind is that the person who is freaking out is temporarily in a lot of trouble and needs some human kindness and reassurance.

1. Put the person in a quiet room away from disturbing noises and lights and curious people. The victim is extremely sensitive to stimulus input and is easily distracted.

2. Feeling that one is losing one's mind is quite common. Reassure the person that this is the drug working and that the feeling will pass when the drug wears off.

3. Depending on what the person took and how strong the dose, you may have to stay with him or her for a few hours. If you go to an emergency room, be prepared to stay the whole time.

4. Do not be judgmental or berate the victim. Speak in a calm and soothing voice. The person who stays with the victim should be someone the victim trusts.

5. Sometimes physical contact can be very important. Holding hands or holding or even gently rocking the victim in your arms can be very reassuring. However, if he is going through some paranoid feelings, he may not want anyone to touch him. Go with the flow.

6. Make the person physically as comfortable as possible—lots of pillows, a blanket, a comfortable chair. Try to restrict the person to that one room. However, as paranoid feelings sometimes include fear of being trapped, you may have to move around the house or apartment with him.

7. Light snacks and beverages are okay. No booze or drugs!

8. Do not leave the victim alone at any time. Stay there and give continuous psychological support.

9. Orient the victim often as to time and place.

10. If it gets rough, have someone help you. You can take turns staying in the room with the victim. Assure the victim that someone will be there at all times.

The pursuit of pleasure by means of drugs can be a risky business. Perhaps someday we will have safer compounds with which to pursue what Carlos Castaneda has called "separate realities." If you are open and honest with yourself about both risks and benefits of drug taking, you can draw your own line between drug use and drug abuse. The difference between short-term pleasures and long-term nightmares is sometimes only a snort, toke, or shot. Remember that most of what you experience while high is simply another aspect of yourself. Drugs may show us things about our inner selves and exaggerate or emphasize them, but they never can put something there that did not already exist. Drugs can delight and instruct or frighten and harm us. The difference depends on how much responsibility you are willing to take about what goes into your body.

Summary of Drug Information

TYPE OF DRUG: STIMULANTS

Amphetaminelike Drugs

Generic names: Amphetamine, benzphetamine, dextroamphetamine, diethylpropion, levamphetamine, methamphetamine, methylphenidate, phendimetrazine, phenmetrazine, phentermine

Brand names: Amodril, Bamadex, Benzedrine, Biphetamine, Desoxyn, Dexedrine, Didrex, Eskatrol, Fastin, Fetamin, Ionamin, Obotan, Obetrol, Plegine, Preludin, Ritalin, Tenuate, Tepanil, Tora, Wilpo

Street names: Bennies, black beauties, copilots, dexies, hearts, meth, pep pills, speed, uppers, ups

Indications: Appetite suppression (anorexics), hyperactivity, fatigue, narcolepsy

Contraindications: During or within 14 days following the administration of monoamine oxidase (MAO) inhibitors (antidepressants). Patients with a history of drug abuse. Patients suffering from severe anxiety or who are in an agitated state. Hyperthyroidism (overactive thyroid disorder). Many of these drugs are also contraindicated for persons with symptomatic cardiovascular disease, glaucoma, advanced arteriosclerosis (hardening of the arteries), being treated for high blood pressure.

Possible side effects and/or adverse reactions: Nervousness, increased heart rate, insomnia, dizziness, headache, tremor, euphoria, dysphoria, dryness of the mouth, unpleasant taste, heart palpitations, rapid or irregular heartbeat. Some serious adverse reactions include alteration of insulin in the management of diabetes, increased blood pressure, changes in libido, sexual impotence, behavioral disturbances, and amphetamine psychosis.

Physical dependency: Yes

Psychological dependency: Yes

Other information: The *PDR* contains the following warning: "Amphetamines have a high potential for abuse. They should thus be tried only in weight reduction programs for patients in whom alternative therapy has not been effective. Administration of amphetamines for prolonged periods of time in obesity may lead to drug dependence and must be avoided. Particular attention should be paid to the possibility of subjects obtaining amphetamines for non-therapeutic use or distribution to others, and the drugs should be prescribed or dispensed sparingly." Safety in pregnancy has not been established. Do not use during breast feeding without discussion with your doctor. Should not be used for more than two weeks for appetite control. Sudden stoppage of the drug can lead to extreme fatigue, mental depression, and sleep disturbance (at high doses). Most of the drugs sold on the street as amphetamines are caffeine or other drug substitutes.

Cocaine

Generic name: Cocaine

Brand name: None. No medical use today. Derived in illicit drug factories from the leaves of *Erythroxylon coca.*

Street names: Bernice, coke, flake, girl, happy dust, lady, snow

Indications: No medical indications. Cocaine stimulates the central nervous system, leading to euphoria, excitation, restlessness, and a feeling of heightened mental and physical power. One of the pleasure drugs associated with sex.

Possible side effects and/or adverse reactions: As dosage increases tremors and convulsions can occur. Overdose is characterized by anxiety, depression, headache, confusion, dry throat, dizziness, and fainting. Although deaths are rare, they can occur from cardiovascular or respiratory collapse. Inflammation of the nasal mucosa, nasal sores, and nasal bleeding are not uncommon when coke is snorted. Cocaine psychosis can occur and is very similar to amphetamine psychosis.

Physical dependency: No

Psychological dependency: Yes

Other information: There is no evidence for physical dependency, but chronic users report a "temporary tolerance" with the high getting shorter. When use is heavy or continuous, a strong psychic dependency occurs. This danger is increased when coke is freebased or injected. Frequent users go through some nasty depressions and craving when they stop. The price can put you into debt rather easily.

Nicotine

Generic name: Nicotine
Brand name: None as such. Found in all tobacco products.
Street name: None
Indications: None. It has been discarded as a therapeutic agent by modern medicine.
Contraindications: Should not be used by anyone with respiratory problems. Smoking increases metabolism in the human body. There is evidence that smoking increases the metabolism of painkillers like Talwin (pentazocine) and Darvon (propoxyphene, phenacetin, etc.) and the asthma medication theophylline (found in Bronkaid, Bronkotabs, Elixophyllin, Marax, Tedral, Quadrinal, etc.). The result is that smokers probably get diminished therapeutic benefits of these drugs.
Possible side effects and/or adverse reactions: Nicotine acts as a stimulant on the heart and nervous system. When tobacco smoke is inhaled, the immediate effects on the body are a faster heartbeat and elevated blood pressure. It also causes users to urinate more frequently. The tars and carbon monoxide cause a long list of serious health problems, including cancer and cardiovascular and respiratory ailments, some of which can result in death.
Physical dependency: Yes
Psychological dependency: Yes
Other information: The risks greatly outweigh the supposed benefits. It's caveat emptor all the way.

Xanthines

Generic names: Caffeine, theobromine, theophylline
Brand names: Caffeine: in coffee, tea, colas (check ingredients), cocoa and chocolate products, and the following prescription medications and OTCs:
APC, Apectol, Buff-A Comp tablets, Butalbital with APC tablets, Cafamine T.D. capsules, Cafergot, Cafergot P-B, Cetased, Efed II, Emprazil,

Esgic, Excedrin, Fiorinal, G-1 capsules, Medigesic Plus, Migral, Migralam, No Doz, Pacaps, Repan, Rogesic, SK-65 Compound, Soma Compound, Synalgos, Synalgos-DC, T-Gesic, Vanquish, Vivarin, Caffedrine capsules, Anacin, Midol, Aqua-ban, Permathene H$_2$O Off, Pre-Mens Forte, Coryban-D, Dristan, Triaminicin, Dexatrim, Dietac, Promaline

Theobromine: in Anthemol, Anthemol-N

Theophyllin: in Accurbron, Aerolate, Aquaphyllin, Azma-Aid, Bronkodyl, Bronkolixir, Bronkotabs, Constant-T, Elixicon, Elixophyllin, Isofil T.D., Isuprel Hydrochloride, LāBID 100 & 250, Marax, Mudrane GG, Physpan, Pulm, Quibron, Respbid, Slo-Phyllin, Somophyllin, Sustaire, Synophylate, TEH, Tedral, Theobid, Theobid Jr., Theoclear L.A., Theo-Dur, Theofedral, Theolair, Theon, Theo-Organidin, Theophedrizine, Theophyl, Theophylline, Theospan, Theostat, Theovent, Quadrinal
Street names: None
Indications: Stimulants, pain relievers, diuretics, cold remedies, weight control aids, asthma relief, arteriosclerosis, etc.
Contraindications: Severe heart disease, active stomach ulcer, allergic reaction to any previous dosage
Possible side effects and/or adverse reactions: nervousness, insomnia, increased urine output, nausea, vomiting, diarrhea, stomach irritation, headaches, heartburn, palpitations, dizziness, confusion, agitation (varies greatly according to dose and individual).
Physical dependency: Caffeine: yes
Psychological dependency: Caffeine: yes
Other information: No stimulant should be substituted for normal sleep where physical alertness is required. The effects of the xanthines are additive and cross-tolerant, when taking medications with xanthines, keep your consumption of such beverages as coffee, tea and colas accordingly low. Experts suggest no more than five cups of coffee per day (as evidence is unclear regarding the safety of caffeine, moderation is the smartest way to go).

TYPE OF DRUG: SEDATIVES

Alcohol

Generic name: Ethyl alcohol or ethanol
Brand names: Many different brands of beer, wine, and liquor. Many people are surprised at the number of medications which contain alcohol.

Some alcohol-containing preparations for coughs, colds, and congestion:

Drug	% of alcohol
Actol Expectorant	1.5
Ambenyl Expectorant	5.0
Calcidrine Syrup	6.0
Chlor-Trimeton Syrup	7.0
Citra Forte Syrup	2.0
Coryban-D Syrup	7.5
Demazin Syrup	7.5
Dilaudid Cough Syrup	5.0
Dimetane Elixir	3.0
Dimetane Expectorant	3.5
Dimetane Expectorant-D.C.	3.5
Dimetapp Elixir	2.3
Hycotuss Expectorant & Syrup	10.0
Lufyllin-GG	17.0
Novahistine DH	5.0
Novahistine DMX	10.0
Novahistine Elixir	5.0
Novahistine Expectorant	7.5
Nyquil Cough Syrup	25.0
Ornacol Liquid	8.0
Periactin Syrup	5.0
Pertussin 8-Hour Syrup	9.5
Phenergan Expectorant, Plain	7.0
Phenergan Expectorant, Codeine	7.0
Phenergan VC Expectorant, Plain	7.0
Phenergan VC Expectorant, Codeine	7.0
Phenergan Expectorant, Pediatric	7.0
Phenergan Syrup Fortis	1.5
Polaramine Expectorant	7.2
Quibron Elixir	15.0
Robitussin	3.5
Robitussin A-C	3.5
Robitussin-PE and -DM	1.4
Robitussin-CF	4.75
Rondec-DM	.6

Drug	% of alcohol
Theo-Organidin Elixir	15.0
Triaminic Expectorant	5.0
Triaminic Expectorant D.H.	5.0
Tussar-2 Syrup	5.0
Tussar SF Syrup	12.0
Tussi-Organidin	15.0
Tuss-Ornade	7.5
Tylenol Elixir	7.0
Tylenol Elixir with Codeine	7.0
Tylenol Drops	7.0
Vicks Formula 44	10.0

Other commonly used drugs containing alcohol:

Drug	% of alcohol
Alurate Elixir	20.0
Anaspaz PB Liquid	15.0
Aromatic Elixir	22.0
Asbron Elixir	15.0
Atarax Syrup	.5
Tincture of Belladonna	67.0
Benadryl Elixir	14.0
Bentyl with Phenobarbitol Syrup	19.0
Cas-Evac	18.0
Carbrital Elixir	18.0
Choledyl Elixir	20.0
Decadron Elixir	5.0
Dexedrine Elixir	10.0
Donnagel	3.8
Donnagel-PG	5.0
Donnatal Elixir	23.0
Dramamine Liquid	5.0
Elixophyllin	20.0
Elixophyllin-KI	10.0
Feosol Elixir	5.0
Gevrabon	18.0
Ipecac Syrup	2.0

SUMMARY OF DRUG INFORMATION

Drug	% of alcohol
Isuprel Comp. Elixir	19.0
Kaochlor S-F	5.0
Kaon Elixir	5.0
Kay Ciel	4.0
Kay Ciel Elixir	4.0
Marax Syrup	5.0
Mellaril Concentrate	3.0
Minocin Syrup	5.0
Modane Liquid	5.0
Nembutal Elixir	18.0
Tincture of Paregoric	45.0
Parelixir	18.0
Parepectolin	.69
Propadrine Elixir	16.0
Serpasil Elixir	12.0
Tedral Elixir	15.0
Temaril Syrup	5.7
Theolixir (Elixir Theophylline)	20.0
Valadol	9.0
Vita-Metrazol Elixir	15.0

Street names: Joy juice, booze, hootch, white lightning, 3.2, vino, and many other localized slang terms

Indications: Ethanol has no specific medical indications. Doctors prefer other sedatives to alcohol. As you can tell from the list above, alcohol is used *in combination* with many drugs. Now you know why some cold remedies give you the rest you need (the sedative effects of the alcohol).

Contraindications: Alcoholics. People with allergic reactions to alcohol. Persons with any number of medical conditions which are aggravated by alcohol—see your physician for further information. Liver disorders top the list. Persons taking disulfiram (Antabuse) must be very alert to alcohol in medicines. So must people taking sedative drugs (effects are additive and supra-additive).

Possible side effects and/or adverse reactions: The headache, upset stomach, and lousy feeling that come with a hangover. Alcohol can dull sensation and impair muscular coordination, memory, and judgment. Taken in larger quantities over a long period of time, alcohol can damage the liver and heart and can cause permanent brain damage. Repeated drinking induces tolerance to the drug's effects and dependence. Withdrawal occurs in dependent persons. Pregnant women should avoid alcohol, as more than 3 ounces per day can lead to fetal alcohol syndrome (FAS).

Physical dependency: Yes

Psychological dependency: Yes

Other information: Alcohol should not be mixed with many other medications. Ask your physician or pharmacist for further information. Driving and operating heavy machinery when drinking can be dangerous.

Barbiturates

Generic names: Amobarbital, butabarbital, phenobarbital, secobarbital, amobarbital with secobarbital

Brand names: Alurate Elixir, Amytal, Buff-A Comp, Buticaps, Butisol, Carbrital, Gustase-Plus, Levsin/Phenobarbital, Levsinex/Phenobarbital Timecaps, Mebaral, Nembutal, Pentobarbitol, Pentothal, Phenobarbital, Plexonal, Secobarbital, Seconal, Sedapap-10, Solfoton, T-Gesic Capsules, Tuinal

Street names: Barbs, goof balls, goofers, bluebirds, blue devils, blue heaven, nimbys, yellow jackets, red devils, reds, double trouble, rainbow, tuies

Indications: Relief of anxiety (benzodiazepine tranquilizers are safer), hypnotic or sleep induction effect (newer nonbarbiturate hypnotics are considered safer), preanesthetic medication, prevention of epileptic seizures

Contraindications: History of porphyria, history of an allergic reaction to any barbiturate drug, drug dependency, marked impairment of liver function, alcoholism

Possible side effects and/or adverse reactions: Drowsiness, lethargy, a sense of mental and physical sluggishness, skin rash, hives, localized swelling of eyelids, face or lips, drug fever, "hangover," dizziness, unsteadiness, nausea, vomiting, diarrhea, paradoxical excitement, respiratory depression, apnea

Physical dependency: Yes

Psychological dependency: Yes

Other information: The use of alcohol or any other sedative drug has an additive effect. Do not plan on doing any mental concentration or driving of a vehicle when using barbiturates. Consult your doctor about drugs which should not be mixed with barbiturates (like coumarin anticoagulants). Some people experience a paradoxical effect when taking barbs as sleep medicine—after 2 to 4 weeks they keep you up instead of putting you to sleep. There is little to recommend barbiturates in the drug scene or in medical circles.

Nonbarbiturates

Generic names: Carbromal, chloral hydrate, ethchlorvynol, ethinamate, flurazepam, glutethimide, methaqualone, methyprylon

Brand names: Ativan injection, Carbrital, Dalmane, Doriden, Dorimide, Equanil, Felsules, Hydroxyzine HCl, Largon, Mepergan Injection, Noctec, Noludar, Parest, Placydil, Phenergan, Quaalude, Remsed, Somnafac, Somnos, Sopor, Unisom Nighttime Sleep-Aid, Valmid

Street names: Ludes, love drug, Qs, quas, quads, 714s, sopers, wallbangers, disco biscuits, CB, Ciba, sleeping pills

Indications: Sleep induction (hypnotic), preoperative sedation, relief of tension or anxiety (low doses)

Contraindications: Pregnancy, nursing, alcoholism, drug abuse history, allergic reaction to any dosage form, patients with hepatic or renal impairment or severe cardiac disease

Possible side effects and/or adverse reactions: Lightheadedness in the upright position, weakness, unsteadiness in stance and gait, headache, "hangover" effect (excessive sedation), numbness and tingling in the arms and legs, indigestion, nausea, vomiting, diarrhea, skin rash

Physical dependency: Yes

Psychological dependency: Yes

Other information: Avoid large doses or continuous use. The nonbarbiturate sedatives may increase the effects of alcohol, other hypnotics, tranquilizers, antihistamines, pain relievers, and narcotic drugs. These drugs can impair mental alertness, reaction time, etc., and should not be taken if you must drive or operate heavy machinery. Sudden stopping can lead to withdrawal—see your doctor about stepping down gradually. Alcohol should be avoided completely for 6 hours before taking these drugs for sleep.

Minor Tranquilizers

Generic names: Chlorazepate, chlordiazepoxide, diazepam, flurazepam, hydroxyzine, lorazepam, meprobamate, oxazepam, prazepam, promazine

Brand names: Tranxene, Librium, Libritabs, SK-Lygen, Librax, Menrium, Valium, Dalmane, Atarax, Vistaril, Equanil, Miltown, Serax, Ativan, Sparine

Street names: The big "V," tranqs, libs, nerve pills, tranks

Indications: Relief of mild to moderate anxiety and nervous tension (without significant sedation), preoperative apprehension, withdrawal symptoms of alcoholism

Contraindications: Known hypersensitivity to these drugs, alcoholism, pregnancy, nursing (speak with your physician), diabetes, glaucoma (narrow-angle type), children under 6 months, psychotic patients

Possible side effects and/or adverse reactions: "Hangover" effect, drowsiness, lethargy, unsteady gait and stance, increase in the blood level of some diabetics, ataxia, changes in libido, tremor, double vision, blurred vision, menstrual irregularities, fainting

Physical dependency: Yes for most

Psychological dependency: Yes

Other information: One of the big problems with tranqs is that they were really intended for periodic management of acute anxiety or tension, but people take them daily—thus developing a functional ("I can't function without the drug") addiction. Tranqs can increase or decrease the effects of many other drugs. For example, Valium can increase the effects of other sedatives, sleep-inducing drugs, tranqs, antidepressants, narcotic drugs, oral anticoagulants of the coumarin family, and antihypertensives. Meprobamate (Dalmane) may decrease the effects of oral anticoagulants, estrogens, and oral contraceptives. Alcohol should be used only with extreme caution. Pregnant women should avoid tranqs. Valium can increase the likelihood of birth defects. Physical dependency can lead to serious withdrawal symptoms if intake is stopped suddenly. Consult your doctor for an appropriate detoxification schedule. As with any other sedative, the operation of a car or heavy machinery may prove dangerous.

Major Tranquilizers (Antipsychotic Drugs)

Generic names: Acetophenazine, butaperazine, chlorpromazine, chlorprothixene, haloperidol, fluphenazine, mesoridazine, perphenazine,

prochlorperazine, thiothixene, thioridazine, trifluoperazine, trifluopro-
mazine

Brand names: Tindal, Repoise, Chlor-PZ, Thorazine, Tranzine, Pro-
mapar, Taractan, Haldol, Permitil, Prolixin, Lidanar, Serentil, Trilafon,
Compazine, Navane, Mellaril, Stelazine, Vesprin

Street names: None

Indications: Restoration of emotional calm, relief of severe anxiety,
agitation, and psychotic behavior. Antiemetic (antinausea) effect

Contraindications: Varies from drug to drug and includes: allergic
reaction to any dosage form, severe heart disease, Parkinson's disease,
mental depression, bone marrow disorder, very young children, comatose states, presence of large amounts of central nervous system depressants (alcohol, barbiturates, narcotics), heavy use of alcohol

Possible side effects and/or adverse reactions: The phenothiazines
(e.g., Thorazine) can cause a condition known as tardive dyskinesia
with muscle spasms affecting the jaw, neck, back, hands, and feet. Facial
twitching, tongue clicking and the like. Discolored urine (may be of
no consequence), drowsiness, change in libido, dryness of the mouth,
nasal congestion, impaired urination, lethargy, blurred vision, constipation, skin rash

Physical dependency: No

Psychological dependency: Yes

Other information: Although used to combat psychosis, these drugs
are taken by many people as major tranquilizers to cope with minor
psychological problems. They are used to a great extent in nursing
homes. Safety has not been established in pregnancy. Ask your doctor
for guidance concerning breast feeding. It is a good idea not to take
these drugs over long periods of time. A "drug holiday" is a good
way to see how you can cope without the drugs. This should only be
done in cooperation with your doctor. These major tranqs can put a
real crimp in your sex life. Mixed with alcohol these drugs can quickly
lead to oversedation. Withdrawal from these drugs should be gradual.

Phencyclidine

Generic name: Phencyclidine

Brand name: Serynl, Sernylan (these are animal tranquilizers)

Street names: PCP, angel dust, hog, killer weed (KW), dust, TAC,
TIC, erth, green, sheets

Indication: None in humans. Used as a veterinary anesthetic and

tranquilizer. Used only as an illicit drug for its mind-altering effects.
Contraindications: None—not used as medicine for humans. However, any illicit use causing an allergic reaction to any dose form should not be repeated.

Possible side effects and/or adverse reactions: Low doses cause loss of inhibition. Higher doses produce an excited, confused intoxification which can include any of the following: muscle rigidity, loss of concentration and memory, visual disturbances, delirium, feelings of isolation and paranoia, convulsions, speech impairment, violent behavior, fear of death, and changes in body perception. The toxic psychosis that can be induced by PCP closely resembles schizophrenia.

Physical dependency: No

Psychological dependency: Yes. Tolerance to psychic effects is reported by chronic users, and psychological dependence described as craving is reported.

Other information: This drug is quite volatile and can affect different users in vastly disparate ways ranging from withdrawal to severe agitation. Even experienced users cannot be certain how it will affect them each time. Often sprinkled over oregano or parsley and smoked, it is also found sprinkled on marijuana or as a bogus marijuana substitute. Cheap and easy to make and sells for less than grass on the street. A derivative of PCP called Ketamine is now becoming popular.

TYPE OF DRUG: OPIATES AND SYNTHETIC NARCOTICS

Generic names: Heroin, hydromorphone, meperidine, methadone, morphine, opium

Brand names: Dilaudid, Demerol, Adanon, Dolophine (no medical use of heroin)

Street names: H, junk, smack, horse, scag, shit, dollies, M, morph, Miss Emma, dreamer, O, Op, black stuff, meth

Indications: Relief of moderate to severe pain, detoxification from opiate drugs, methadone maintenance therapy, preoperative medication, support of anesthesia, obstetrical analgesia

Contraindications: History of opiate drug abuse, hypersensitivity to any of these drugs, patients using MAO inhibitors, using antihypertensive drugs

Possible side effects and/or adverse reactions: All of these drugs are highly addicting, with tolerance and withdrawal syndromes. Respiratory and circulatory depression, lightheadedness, dizziness, nausea, vomiting, sweating, dry mouth, constipation, lowered libido, visual disturbance, uncoordinated muscle movements, weakness, euphoria

Physical dependency: Yes

Psychological dependency: Yes

Other information: Chronic users who inject these drugs run the risks of embolism, hepatitis, sores, abscesses, blood poisoning, inflammation and collapse of veins, congestion of the lungs, and pneumonia. Opiate habits become very expensive and often lead to a criminal lifestyle to support the habit. Heroin and other opiates are a real sexual downer. Use of any of these drugs with other CNS depressants can result in serious oversedation. Science is still searching for an effective nonaddicting painkiller.

TYPE OF DRUG: ANTIDEPRESSANTS

Mono-amine Oxidase (MAO) Inhibitors

Generic names: Flurazolidone, iproniazid, isocarboxazid, mebanazine, nialamide, pargyline, phenelzine, pheniprazine, phenoxypropazine, piohydrazine, tranylcypromine

Brand names: Actomol, Adapin, Catron, Drazine, Eutonyl, Furoxone, Marplan, Marsilid, Nardil, Niamid, Parnate, Tersavid

Street names: None

Indications: Gradual relief of emotional depression and lifting of mood, usually used when depressed patients are not responsive to tricyclic antidepressant drugs.

Contraindications: Ever had an allergic reaction, advanced heart disease, impaired liver function or disease; taking any other antidepressant drugs or sympathomimetic drugs (such as amphetamines, dopamine, epinephrine, etc.); excessive amounts of caffeine, foods containing tryptophan (broad beans) or tyramine (cheese, beers, wines, pickled herring, chicken livers, yeast extract, etc.).

Possible side effects and/or adverse reactions: Vary from drug to drug and include: insomnia, lightheadedness, dizziness, weakness, feeling of impending faint in the upright position (orthostatic hypotension), blurred vision, muscle twitching, vertigo, headache, tremors, impaired memory. Sexual dysfunction including impotence, problems with urination, impaired ejaculation in men, and delayed orgasm in women. Incompatible with many other medications (including many OTCs) and certain foods.

Physical dependency: No

Psychological dependency: Possible

Other information: MAO inhibitor antidepressants are used mainly when the tricyclics are either contraindicated or ineffective. When used carefully with a restricted diet they can help. Tricyclics are preferred because they have milder side effects. Severe dietary restrictions are necessary so that hypertensive episodes, which can lead to a stroke, do not occur. These drugs are real sexual downers.

Tricyclic Antidepressants

Generic names: amitriptyline, clomipramine, desipramine, doxepin, imipramine, nortriptyline, opipramol, protriptyline, trimipramine

Brand names: Anafranil, Aventyl, Elavil, Ensidon, Norpramin, Pertofrane, Presamine, Sinequan, Surmontil, Tofranil, Vivactil, Amitryl, Endep, Etrafon, Limbitrol, Triavil, Antipress, Imavate, Janimine, Pamelor, Adapin

Street names: None

Indication: Gradual improvement of mood and relief of emotional depression

Contraindications: glaucoma (narrow-angle type), ever had an allergic reaction, taking or have taken an MAO inhibitor within the last 14 days, recovering from a recent heart attack, child under 12 years of age

Possible side effects and/or adverse reactions: Dry mouth, blurred vision, constipation, urinary retention, drowsiness, eye pain, irregular heartbeat, fainting, shakiness, increased appetite for sweets

Physical dependency: No

Psychological dependency: Rare

Other information: Drowsiness should disappear after a few weeks but driving can be hazardous during this early period. People find that if they stand up slowly the dizziness is reduced. Patience is required as it may take up to 6 weeks for all benefits to be experienced (about 70% of patients get them).

TYPE OF DRUG: MARIJUANA AND ITS COUSINS

Generic name: Cannabis sativa is the hemp plant, from which marijuana is derived. There are roughly 360-odd chemicals in the cannabis plant. Delta-9-tetrahydrocannabinol (THC) is one of a total of 61 canna-binoids found in the plant and is the one that gets you stoned and probably is responsible for the "munchies" (powerful hunger induced by smoking strong marijuana). There are powerful cousins to marijuana grown in other parts of the world such as ganja (Jamaica) and bhang (India). Marijuana is only one-tenth as strong as hashish, which is the pure resin of the plant.

Brand names: Not commercially marketed. With special permission physicians may prescribe THC for certain conditions.

Street names: Pot, grass, mary jane, weed, smoke, shit, reefer, hemp, herb, thai stick, dope, ganja, hash oil, m.j., stuff

Indication: Used to treat some forms of glaucoma and as an anti-emetic (antinausea) drug for the reaction to cancer treatment.

Contraindications: Allergic reaction to cannabis products, hypersen-sitivity to the drugs contained in marijuana, respiratory ailments (which prevent smoking), history of drug abuse. The effects of marijuana on growing young bodies are not known at this time. Grass may contain carcinogenic elements (this too is not yet known for sure).

Possible side effects and/or adverse reactions: Euphoria, dry mouth and throat, "munchies," disorientation, difficulty in concentration, com-pulsive talking ("motor mouth"), giggling and hysteria, altered sense of time, increased heart rate (usually subsides), reddening of the eyes, altered sense of body image, acute panic anxiety reaction, and very rarely a marijuana-induced psychosis

Physical dependency: No

Psychological dependency: Possible

Other information: Safety in pregnancy has not been established; women are advised not to smoke at all during pregnancy. A lot more research is needed on the long-term effect of marijuana use. Effect of drug will depend on set, setting, and THC content. Beware of adulterants like paraquat, fungal growths, salmonella, and PCP.

TYPE OF DRUG: HALLUCINOGENS

Generic names: Mescaline, psilocybin, lysergic acid diethylamide (LSD), dimethyltriptamine (DMT), 2,5 dimethoxy-4-methylamphet-amine (STP), methylenedioxyamphetamine (MDA)

Brand names: None. Illicit hallucinogens are sold under a wide vari-ety of street names.

Street names: LSD: acid, cubes, "25," Lucy in the Sky with Diamonds (from the song by the Beatles); some street "brands" have included blotter, blue cheer, microdots, sunshine, windowpane, white lightning, chocolate chip, clear light

Mescaline: buttons, divine cactus, peyote

Psilocybin: flesh of the gods, magic mushroom, sacred mushroom

DMT: lunch-hour trip, businessman's trip

STP (DOM): serenity, tranquility and peace

Indications: No medical indications at this time. Research with LSD in the treatment of alcoholism and mental illness has stopped. Some of the hallucinogens (also called psychedelics) such as peyote and ganja are used in religious rituals.

Contraindications: Allergic reactions or hypersensitivity to these drugs, emotional instability, medicines and other drugs that can cause adverse reactions, great fear of these drugs

Possible side effects and/or adverse reactions: The infamous "bad trip" with exaggerated body distortion, fear of death, going insane, or being abandoned—generally any bad reaction to the altered perceptions caused by hallucinogens. Usual effects are changes in sensation, depth perception, passage of time, body image. Wide range of emotional reactions is possible. Some people never return from a trip, spending months or longer in a frightening altered state. Flashbacks—re-experiencing the LSD effects without ingesting more acid—can occur. Watch out for bogus drugs when buying on the street.

Physical dependency: No

Psychological dependency: Possible but rare

Other information: For reasons that are not clear, LSD seems to be making a comeback. Perhaps the kids of today think that they missed something from the '60s. These drugs are not to be taken lightly. If someone is on a bad trip, consult Chapter 5 of this book.

TYPE OF DRUG: THE VOLATILE INHALANTS

Generic names: Amyl nitrite, butyl nitrite, isobutyl nitrite
Brand names: Amyl nitrite (Aspirols and Vaporole)

Butyl and isobutyl nitrite: Aroma of Man, Ban Apple, Black Jac, Bolt, Bullet, Cat's Meow, Cum, Dr. Bananas, Gas, Hardware, Heart On,

Hi Baller, Jac Aroma, Krypt Tonight, Loc-a-Roma, Oz, Rush, Satan's Scent, Shotgun, Toilet Water. Most of these are sold as "room odorizers."

Aroma, Krypt Tonight, Loc-a-Roma, Oz, Rush, Satan's Scent, Shotgun, Toilet Water. Most of these are sold as "room odorizers."

Street names: poppers, snappers

Indications: Amyl nitrite is a vasodilator which relaxes smooth muscle so small blood vessel are expanded and blood pressure is lowered. Relief of heart pains associated with angina pectoris, relaxation of sphincter muscles. Butyl has no medical uses.

Contraindications: Allergic reaction to any dose form. Amyl nitrite is available only upon prescription from your doctor. Not described in the 1982 *PDR.*

Possible side effects and/or adverse reactions: Headache, dizziness, accelerated heart rate, nausea, nasal irritation, cough (only the headache tends to persist). Men can lose erection.

Physical dependency: No

Psychological dependency: Possible

Other information: Kids sniff this stuff to get high. Kids and adults use it to experience intensified orgasms during sex. Butyls smell awful. Effects are very short-lived, lasting only minutes. The problem is that you have to stop sexual activity to use this stuff, which can be a real turn-off, especially for women. Don't be fooled: this foul-smelling stuff is anything but a "room odorizer" (its FDA designation). A wide variety of solvents are also sniffed, particularly by kids, in an effort to get high. The table below lists these solvents and some of their physical effects.

Abused Solvents

Volatile Solvent	Physical Effects
1. aromatic hydrocarbons:	
benzene	bone marrow, liver, heart, adrenal, and kidney impairment
xylene	bone marrow impairment
toluene	bone marrow, liver, kidney, and CNS impairment

287

Abused Solvents

Volatile Solvent	Physical Effects
2. aliphatic hydrocarbons:	
hexane	polyneuropathy
naphtha	low toxicity
petroleum distillates	low toxicity
3. halogenated hydrocarbons:	
trichloroethylene	cardiac arrhythmia, kidney, and liver impairment
1,1,1-trichloroethane (methylchloroform	CNS, lung, kidney, cardiac, and pancreas impairment
Carbon tetrachloride	lung, liver, kidney, and CNS impairment
ethylene dichloride	spleen, CNS, liver, and kidney impairment
methylene chloride	CNS, liver, and kidney impairment
4. freons:	
trichlorofluoromethane (FC11)	cardiac arrhythmia
dichloroflouromethane (FC114)	cardiac arrhythmia
cyroflurane	cardiac arrhythmia
dichlorotetraflouromethane (FC12)	cardiac arrhythmia
5. ketones:	
acetone	low toxicity
cyclohexanone	
methylethylketone	peripheral neuropathy, pulmonary hypertension
methylisobutylketone	peripheral neuropathy
methylbutylketone	peripheral neuropathy
methylamylketone	peripheral neuropathy
6. esters:	
ethyl acetate	liver and kidney impairment
amyl acetate	low toxicity
butyl acetate	low toxicity

Abused Solvents

Volatile Solvent	Physical Effects
7. alcohols:	
methyl alcohol	optic atrophy
isopropyl alcohol	low toxicity
8. glycols:	
methyl cellulose acetate	liver and kidney impairment
ethylene glycol	liver, kidney, lung, and CNS impairment
9. gasoline, leaded	lung, bone marrow, liver, CNS, and peripheral nerve impairment

Source: S. Cohen "Inhalants and Solvents," Chapter in *Youth Drug Abuse: Problems, Issues, and Treatment,* ed. G. M. Beschner and A. S. Friedman. Lexington, Mass.: Lexington Books, 1979, p. 287.

APPENDIX B:

Additional Readings

Ernest L. Abel. *Marihuana, The First Twelve Thousand Years.* McGraw-Hill Book Company, New York, 1982.
Well written and fascinating. Compresses a great deal of historical information into a paperback. A must for understanding marijuana from a historical frame of reference. Scholarly but easy to read.

Alcoholics Anonymous World Services, Inc. *Alcoholics Anonymous—the story of how many thousands of men and women have recovered from alcoholism.* New York: Alcoholics Anonymous World Services, Inc., 1976.
Known as the "Big Book," it is the definitive text on A.A. Excellent source book for students and those who are members. For those looking for practical information, the book *Living Sober* published by the same folks is about 450 pages shorter.

American Pharmaceutical Association. *Handbook of Nonprescription Drugs,* 5th ed. Washington, D.C.: American Pharmaceutical Association, 1977.
People who are into OTCs will find this expensive ($20) book quite objective and straightforward. Gives an overview of many medicines and tells you the ingredients in many products. Geared for the pharmacist, but can be read by the layman with a dictionary handy. If Joe Graedon recommends it, it must be good.

Baker, Charles E., Jr. *Physicians' Desk Reference.* 36 ed. Oradell, N.J.: Medical Economics Company, Inc., 1982.
This is the physician's "bible" when it comes to prescribing medication. The drug manufacturers pay to place their product information in this tome. It is over 2000 pages in length and contains information on approximately 2000 products. Contains 38 pages of color plates to help you identify various products. Products are indexed by name, category, generic and chemical name, diagnostic information. Also contains a list of poison control centers and a guide to management of drug overdose. Cost is high, about $19.95 in

most bookstores. For less expensive and easier-to-read books with similar (but not as comprehensive) information see Long, Graedon, and Silverman. This *PDR* deals only with prescription medications. The same publisher also has created a *PDR* for nonprescription drugs and a *PDR* for ophthalmology.

Beschner, George M., and Alfred S. Friedman. *Youth Drug Abuse: Problems, Issues and Treatment.* Lexington, Mass.: Lexington Books, 1979.
This 681-page compendium of writings and research on the youth drug scene is not for the beginner unless you are willing to wade through a lot of statistical material. Excellent reference source for serious students of the subject. Dr. David Smith, Diane Striar, and I wrote a nonstatistical chapter on treatment services for youthful drug users.

Blaine, Rabbi Allan. *Alcoholism and the Jewish Community.* New York: Commission on Synagogue Relations, Federation of Jewish Philanthropies of New York, 1980.
Compendium of writings scratching the surface of a long-denied phenomena: the alcoholic who is a Jew. Contains a general overview, a Jewish historical perspective, studies on Jewish alcoholism, the role of home, family, and community, the role of the rabbi and the synagogue. Ellen Bayer and I wrote a chapter about the first spiritual retreat for Jewish alcoholics. A good source book for the beginner.

Brecher, Edward M., and the Editors of *Consumer Reports. Licit and Illicit Drugs.* Boston: Little, Brown and Company, 1972.
An excellent primer for those who are new to the drug scene. Contains an extensive amount of interesting historical material on a wide variety of drugs—caffeine, narcotics, amphetamines, barbiturates, inhalants, LSD, marijuana, and hashish. The authors arrive at some unique and unorthodox conclusions and make some startling recommendations for policies governing treatment and prevention of drug abuse.

Bush, Patricia J. *Drugs, Alcohol and Sex.* New York: Richard Marek Publishers, 1980.
Pulls together a wide literature into a cohesive text. Examines the effects of many different classes of drugs—street, prescription, OTC. Dr. Bush collected specific data on drugs and sex from 250 people and compares their statements with findings in the literature. Excellent sections of aphrodisiacs and placebo effects.

The Editors of *Consumer Reports. The Medicine Show,* rev. ed. Mount Vernon, N.Y.: Consumers Union, 1979.
The subtitle is "Some plain truths about popular remedies for common ailments." This is a wonderfully objective and informative book which covers a wide range of illnesses, conditions, and drugs. Debunks wonder and miracle drugs. Can be obtained from Consumer Report Books, Dept. AA10, P.O. Box 350, Orangeburg, New York, 10962.

Freudenberger, Herbert J., and Geraldine Richelson. *Burn-Out: the High Cost of High Achievement.* Garden City, N.Y.: Doubleday & Company, Anchor Press, 1980.
Explains one of the major reasons why people try to anesthetize and tranquilize themselves with drugs. Particularly relevant to the subject of drugs in the workplace. Easy reading but extremely thought-provoking.

Gordon, Barbara. *I'm Dancing as Fast as I Can.* New York: Harper & Row, 1979.
One woman's nightmare with the drug Valium. Shows how sudden stopping of a drug can lead to serious withdrawal reactions, including mental breakdown. Moving story of Ms. Gordon's struggle to recover.

Graedon, Joe. *The People's Pharmacy—2.* New York: Avon Books, 1980.
This is the second book in a series (first one was entitled *The People's Pharmacy*). Joe Graedon may be the best friend that the American public has when it comes to prescription and OTC drugs. His informative style is delivered with honesty and humor. He lays all the sacred cows to rest and helps us to understand how our best protection is information, which he supplies in abundance. *The People's Pharmacy* should be in every home in America. Some of the sections in the book include drug interactions, for women only, vitamins, drugs and your head, drugs and children, drugs and older people, and saving money in the pharmacy.

Hastings, Arthur C., James Fadiman, and James S. Gordon, eds. *The Complete Guide to Holistic Medicine—Health for the Whole Person.* New York: Bantam Books, 1980.
Encyclopedic in scope, this paperback is a wonderful introduction to holistic medicine. It serves as an excellent overview to the subject without losing a sense of objectivity. It can help you to see that your own responsibilities for your health are within your grasp. But you will require new ways of looking at yourself. Deals with everything from foods as medicine to death and dying.

Johnson, Lloyd D., Jerald G. Bachman, and Patrick M. O'Malley. *Highlights from Student Drug Use in America, 1975–1980.* The University of Michigan, Institute for Social Research and the National Institute on Drug Abuse. Available from the Alcohol, Drug Abuse, and Mental Health Administration, Printing and Publications Management Branch, 5600 Fishers Lane (Rm.6C–02), Rockville, Maryland 20857.
Excellent source material on student drug use and drug trends during this five-year period. Useful for comparing localities with national trends. Contains a lot of statistics, charts, and graphs.

Knowles, John, ed. *Doing Better and Feeling Worse: Health in the United States.* New York: W. W. Norton, 1977.
Carefully spells out the importance of individual responsibility for our health. Also explores political, technological, and fiscal realities of health care in a time when nearly 10 percent of our GNP is spent on health. Strong emphasis on health maintenance as opposed to "fix it when it breaks down" approach.

Lingeman, Richard R. *Drugs from A to Z: A Dictionary.* 2nd ed. New York: McGraw-Hill Book Company, 1974.
Still timely. A great introduction to the mysterious-sounding jargon of the street drug scene with entries from the world of medicine as well. Now you can learn just what your children are talking about when they use terms like lids, jay, lady, buzz, etc.

Long, James W. *The Essential Guide to Prescription Drugs—What You Need to Know for Safe Drug Use.* New York: Harper and Row, 1980.
Available as a large paperback at half the price of the *PDR*. Well written and easy for the lay person to understand. It contains information on 212 generic drugs (1466 brand names) in the form of drug profiles; many useful tables of drug information such as drug interactions, pregnancy, photosensitivity, sleep, alcohol, mood, etc. Clearly defines drug terminology and uses a very straightforward format. Book is indexed by brand and generic names.

ADDITIONAL READINGS

Marin, Peter, and Alan Y. Cohen. *Understanding Drug Use—An Adult's Guide to Drugs and the Young.* New York: Harper & Row, 1971.
The authors provide parents of adolescents with perceptive insights into their children and the drug scene. Has a realistic focus and, unlike many other books on the subject, expresses an affection and respect for adolescents. While some specifics may be out of date, the emphasis on people and not drugs is illuminating.

Martin, James K. and Mark Lender. *Drinking in America.* Free Press-Macmillan, 1982.
A historical review of drinking behavior in America from Colonial times to date. Objective and unbiased, it avoids the emotional traps and gives a vivid and humorous account of the 200 years of warfare between wets and drys.

Rubinstein, Morton K. *A Doctor's Guide to Non-Prescription Drugs.* New York: Signet Books, 1977.
A thought-provoking and extremely practical guide. Book is organized by type of illness or condition, making it easy for you to look up drugs by complaint. Contains a lot of educational material about what to take and not to take. Has loads of information about combination drugs. Inexpensive paperback.

Russianoff, Penelope, ed. *Women in Crisis.* New York: Human Sciences Press, 1981.
The proceedings of the first annual Women in Crisis Conference held in New York City in 1979. Contains seven articles directly on women and drugs, including my own on sexism in drug abuse treatment. Entire book is well done and informative. Must reading for those who act as advocates for women.

Sandmaier, Marian. *The Invisible Alcoholics—Women and Alcohol Abuse in America.* New York: McGraw-Hill Book Company, 1980.
One of the best books available on the subject of women and alcohol. Written by the former Director of Women's Programs for the National Clearinghouse for Alcohol Information and Chair of the National Women's Health Network's Alcoholism Policy Committee.

Scher, Jordan M., ed. *Drug Abuse in Industry: Growing Corporate Dilemma.* Springfield, Ill.: Charles C. Thomas, 1973.
Good introduction to basic concerns of drug use in the workplace. Quality of articles varies greatly but gives an excellent first exposure to a complicated issue. My study of drug-related crime in business and industry appears in this volume.

Selye, Hans. *Stress without Distress.* New York: Signet Books, 1974.
Learn about the scientific nature of human stress. Better than the pop psychology books on the same subject. Selye has an interesting philosophy for living as well as being *the* expert on stress.

Silverman, Harold, and Gilbert Simon. *The Pill Book—The Illustrated Guide to the Most Prescribed Drugs in the United States.* New York: Bantam Books, 1979.
Contains 21 pages of color illustrations of medications. Deals with the 1000 most commonly prescribed drugs with information about drug properties, dosages, side effects, and adverse effects. Has sections on how drugs work, drugs and food, 20 questions to ask about medicine, and other points to remember for safe drug use. Easy to read, inexpensive paperback.

Spotts, James V., and Franklin C. Shontz. *Cocaine Users—A Representative Case Approach.* New York: The Free Press, 1980.
An intensive study of nine different users of cocaine. Background section provides a good introduction to history, pharmacological and physiological actions, and social usage patterns and effects of the drug. Strong emphasis on context and lifestyle of cocaine use.

Weil, Andrew. *The Natural Mind—A New Way of Looking at Drugs and the Higher Consciousness.* Boston: Houghton Mifflin Company, 1972.
One of the most innovative and exciting books on drug use ever written. Goes beyond many stereotypes to explore drug use as a natural pursuit of altered states of consciousness. Easy to read and understand, it will stimulate your thinking about many establishment blind spots about drug use. Explores an interesting dichotomy between "stoned" and "straight" thinking. Dr. Weil is a Harvard-trained physician who provides new ways of thinking about a problem that has divided our nation.

Wolfe, Sidney M., Christopher M. Coley, and the Health Research Group. *Pills That Don't Work—A Consumers' and Doctors' Guide to Over 600 Prescription Drugs That Lack Evidence of Effectiveness.* Farrar, Straus, Giroux: New York, 1980.
We all need this one because the Food and Drug Administration keeps on dragging its feet. The book carefully explains the various categories of drug effectiveness (or lack of same), and then lists over 600 drugs which have failed to meet these definitions but are still on the market. Fascinating reading about a real rip-off.

Where to Get Help

You can obtain educational materials from the following agencies of the Federal Government:

National Clearinghouse for Drug Abuse Information
5600 Fishers Lane, Room 10A–56
Rockville, Maryland 20857

National Clearinghouse for Alcohol Information
Box 2345
Rockville, Maryland 20850

Technical Information Center
Office on Smoking and Health
5600 Fishers Lane, Room 1–16
Rockville, Maryland 20857

National Clearinghouse for Mental Health Information
National Institute of Mental Health
5600 Fishers Lane, Room 11A–33
Rockville, Maryland 20857

National directories of drug abuse and alcoholism treatment programs are available at a nominal cost from:

Superintendent of Documents
U.S. Government Printing Office
Washington, D.C. 20402

Programs are listed by counties within states. In addition, most states have what the federal government has designated as a Single State Agency responsible for drug and alcohol matters. In some states the two are combined, while in others they are separate agencies. Contact your state government for further information.

Information on alcoholism is also available from:

National Council on Alcoholism (NCA)
733 Third Avenue
New York, New York 10017

There exist local affiliates of NCA in most major cities across America. Contact the central office listed above for further information.

For information on Alcoholics Anonymous meetings in your area as well as a variety of pamphlets on A.A.'s philosophy and program, contact:

Alcoholics Anonymous World Services
P.O. Box 459
Grand Central Station
New York, New York 10017
You can usually find an A.A. office in most major cities; contact them for local meeting information.

Al-Anon sponsors self-help groups for spouses, children and other relatives of alcoholics and also has local offices listed in your phone directory. The address for their central office in New York is:

Al-Anon Family Group Headquarters
P.O. Box 182
Madison Square Station
New York, New York 10010

The National Institute of Mental Health has prepared a fact sheet on mutual self-help groups for consumers. It is available at no charge from:

> The Consumer Information Center
> Department 609K
> Pueblo, Colorado 81009

Directories of mutual-help groups are also available from:

> National Self-Help Clearinghouse
> 33 West 42nd Street
> Room 1227
> New York, New York 10036

For further information on the Toughlove program write to:

> Toughlove
> Post Office Box 70
> Sellersville, Pennsylvania 18960

To find out more about poisons in the home, send a stamped, self-addressed envelope to:

> Mr. Anthony DiMarco
> New York City Poison Control Project
> Bellevue Hospital Center
> 27th Street and First Avenue
> New York, N.Y. 10016

APPENDIX D:

The Marijuana Laws

State & Statute	Amount	Possession: 1st Offense	Possession: 2nd Offense	Cultivation	Sale
Alabama	Up to 2.2 lbs. for personal use	0–1 yr. & $1000	2–15 yrs. & $25,000	2–15 yrs. & $25,000	2–15 yrs. & $25,000
20-2-2 20-2-23 20-2-70 20-2-80	Up to 2.2 lbs. not for personal use	2–15 yrs. & $25,000	2–30 yrs. & $50,000	2–15 yrs. & $25,000	2–15 yrs. & $25,000
	2.2–2000 lbs.	5–15 yrs. & $25,000	3–30 yrs. & $50,000	3–15 yrs. & $25,000	3–15 yrs. & $25,000
	2000–10,000 lbs.	5–15 yrs. & $50,000	5–30 yrs. & $100,000	5–15 yrs. & $50,000	5–15 yrs. & $50,000
	More than 10,000 lbs.	15 years & $200,000	15–30 yrs. & $400,000	15 yrs. & $200,000	15 yrs. & $200,000
Alaska	Any amount for private personal use in home	Legal	Legal	Legal	n/a
	Any amount for personal use not in a public place	$0–100	$0–100	$0–100	n/a
17.10.010	Up to 1 oz. in public	$0–100	$0–100	$0–100	n/a
	Smoking marijuana in public	$0–1000	$0–1000	n/a	n/a
through 17.12.150	More than 1 oz. in public for personal use	$0–1000	$0–1000	n/a	n/a

299

State & Statute	Amount	Possession: 1st Offense	Possession: 2nd Offense	Cultivation	Sale
Alaska (cont.)	Any amount for personal use in car or plane or by a person under 18 yrs.	$0–1000	$0–1000	$0–1000	n/a
Arizona 36–1001 36–1002. 05 & 06	More than 1 oz. not for personal use	0–25 yrs. & $20,000	0–life & $25,000	0–25 yrs. & $25,000	0–25 yrs. & $25,000
	Any amount	1½ yrs. & $0–150,000	1½–3 yrs. & $0–150,000	1½ yrs. & $0–150,000	7 yrs. & $150,000
Arkansas 82.2601	Up to 1 oz.	0–1 yr. & $1000	0–5 yrs. & $10,000	2–10 yrs. & $10,000	2–10 yrs. & $10,000
82.2614 82.2617 41.901	Over 1 oz. (Rebuttable presumption of intent to deliver)	2–10 yrs. & $10,000	2–10 yrs. & $10,000	2–10 yrs. & $10,000	2–10 yrs. & $10,000
California Health & Safety Code 11357 thru 11360	Up to 1 oz.	$0–100	$0–100	$0–100	2–4 yrs.
	Over 1 oz.	0–6 mos. & $500	0–6 mos. & $500	16 mos.–3 yrs.	2–4 yrs.
Colorado 12.22.403 12.22.412	Up to 1 oz. not in public	$0–100	$0–100	1–14 yrs. & $1000	1–14 yrs. & $1000

State & Statute	Amount	Possession: 1st Offense	Possession: 2nd Offense	Cultivation	Sale
Colorado (cont.)	Up to 1 oz. in public	0–15 days & $100	0–15 days & $100	1–14 yrs. & $1000	1–14 yrs. & $1000
	More than 1 oz.	0–1 yr. & $500	Probation–2 yrs. & $500–1000	1–14 yrs. & $1000	1–14 yrs. & $1000
Connecticut	Less than 4 oz.	0–1 yr. & $1000	0–5 yrs. & $3000	0–2 yrs. & $1000	0–7 yrs. & $1000
19.443 19.480 19.481	Over 4 oz.	0–5 yrs. & $2000	0–10 yrs. & $5000	0–2 yrs. & $1000	0–7 yrs. & $1000
19.480A 19.450A	More than 2.2 lbs.	0–5 yrs. & $2000	0–10 yrs. & $5000	5–20 yrs.	5–20 yrs.
Delaware 16.4701 16.4714 16.4752 through 16.4754	Any amount	0–2 yrs. & $500	0–7 yrs. & $500	0–10 yrs. & $1000–10,000	0–10 yrs. & $1000–10,000
Florida 893.02 893.13	Up to 20 grams	0–1 yr. & $1000	0–1 yr. & $1000	0–5 yrs. & $5000	0–5 yrs. & $5000
through 16.4754	20 grams–100 lbs.	0–5 yrs. & $5000	0–5 yrs. & $5000	0–5 yrs. & $5000	0–5 yrs. & $5000
	100–2000 lbs.	3–30 yrs. & $25,000	3–30 yrs. & $25,000	3–30 yrs. & $25,000	3–30 yrs. & $25,000
	2000–10,000 lbs.	5–30 yrs. & $50,000	5–30 yrs. & $50,000	5–30 yrs. & $50,000	5–30 yrs. & $50,000

State & Statute	Amount	Possession: 1st Offense	Possession: 2nd Offense	Cultivation	Sale
Florida (cont.)	Over 10,000 lbs.	15–30 yrs. & $200,000	15–30 yrs. & $200,000	15–30 yrs. & $200,000	15–30 yrs. & $200,000
Georgia 79A.802 79A.811	Up to 1 oz.	0–1 yr. & $1000	1–10 yrs.	1–10 yrs.	1–10 yrs.
79A.9917	1 oz.–100 lbs.	1–10 yrs.	1–10 yrs.	1–10 yrs.	1–10 yrs.
	100–2000 lbs.	5–10 yrs. & $25,000	5–10 yrs. & $25,000	5–10 yrs. & $25,000	5–10 yrs. & $25,000
	2000–10,000 lbs.	7–10 yrs. & $50,000	7–10 yrs. & $50,000	7–10 yrs. & $50,000	7–10 yrs. & $50,000
	More than 10,000 lbs.	15 yrs. & $200,000	15 yrs. & $200,000	15 yrs. & $200,000	15 yrs. & $200,000
Hawaii 712.1240 712.1249	Up to 1 oz.	0–30 days & $500	0–30 days & $500	0–30 days & $500	0–1 yr. & $1000
706.640	1–2 oz.	0–1 yr. & $1000	0–1 yr. & $1000	0–1 yr. & $1000	0–1 yr. & $1000
	2 oz.–2.2 lbs.	0–1 yr. & $1000	0–1 yr. & $1000	0–1 yr. & $1000	0–5 yrs. & $5000
	More than 2.2 lbs.	0–5 yrs. & $5000	0–5 yrs. & $5000	0–5 yrs. & $5000	0–5 yrs. & $5000

State & Statute	Amount	Possession: 1st Offense	Possession: 2nd Offense	Cultivation	Sale
Idaho 37.2701 37.2705	Up to 3 oz.	0–1 yr. & $1000	0–2 yrs. & $2000	0–5 yrs. & $15,000	0–5 yrs. & $15,000
37.2732	More than 3 oz.	0–5 yrs. & $10,000	0–10 yrs. & $20,000	0–5 yrs. & $15,000	0–5 yrs. & $15,000
Illinois 56.5.703 through	Up to 2.5 grams	0–30 days & $500	0–30 days & $500	0–6 mos. & $500	0–6 mos. & $500
56.5.705 38.1005 8.1,9.1	2.5–10 grams	0–6 mos. & $500	0–6 mos. & $500	0–1 yr. & $1000	0–1 yr. & $1000
	10–30 grams	0–1 yr. & $1000	1–3 yrs. & $10,000	1–3 yrs. & $10,000	1–3 yrs. & $10,000
	30–500 grams	1–3 yrs. & $10,000	2–5 yrs. & $10,000	2–5 yrs. & $10,000	2–5 yrs. & $10,000
	Over 500 grams	2–5 yrs. & $10,000	2–5 yrs. & $10,000	3–7 yrs. & $10,000	3–7 yrs. & $10,000
Indiana 35.48.1.1 35.48.2.4 35.48.4. 10–12	Up to 30 grams	0–1 yr. & $5000	0–2 yrs. & $10,000	0–1 yr. & $5000	0–1 yr. & $5000
	More than 30 grams	0–2 yrs. & $10,000	0–2 yrs. & $10,000	0–2 yrs. & $10,000	0–2 yrs. & $10,000
Iowa 204.101 204.204	Any amount	0–6 mos. & $1000	0–18 mos. & $3000		

State & Statute	Amount	Possession: 1st Offense	Possession: 2nd Offense	Cultivation	Sale
204.401 204.410 204.411	Under 1 oz.			0–6 mos. & $1000	0–6 mos. & $1000
	Over 1 oz.			0–5 yrs. & $1000	0–5 yrs. & $1000
Kansas 65.4101 65.4105 65.4127B 21.4501 through 21.4503	Any amount	0–1 yr. & $2500	1–10 yrs. & $5000	0–1 yr. & $2500	1–20 yrs. & $10,000
Kentucky 218A.010 218A.050 218A.990	Any amount	0–90 days & $250	0–90 days & $250	0–1 yr. & $500	0–1 yr. & $500
Louisiana 40.961 40.964 40.967	Up to 100 lbs.	0–6 mos. & $500	0–5 yrs. & $2000	0–10 yrs. & $15,000	0–10 yrs. & $15,000
	100–2000 lbs.	5–10 yrs. & $25,000	5–10 yrs. & $25,000	5–10 yrs. & $25,000	5–10 yrs. & $25,000
	2000–10,000 lbs.	10–15 yrs. & $50,000	10–15 yrs. & $50,000	10–15 yrs. & $50,000	10–15 yrs. & $50,000
	More than 10,000 lbs.	15–20 yrs. & $200,000	15–20 yrs. & $200,000	15–20 yrs. & $200,000	15–20 yrs. & $200,000

State & Statute	Amount	Possession: 1st Offense	Possession: 2nd Offense	Cultivation	Sale
Maine 17A.1107 through 17A.1103	Up to 1½ oz. for personal use	$0–200	$0–200	$0–200	n/a
17A.1106 22.2383	1½ oz.–2 lbs.	(presumed to be for sale)		0–1 yr. & $1000	0–1 yr. & $1000
	2 to 1000 lbs.	(presumed to be for sale)		0–5 yrs. & $2500	0–5 yrs. & $2500
	More than 1000 lbs.	(presumed to be for sale)		0–10 yrs. & $10,000	0–10 yrs. & $10,000
Maryland 27.277 27.279 27.286	Any amount for personal use	0–1 yr. & $1000	0–2 yrs. & $2000	0–1 yr. & $1000	n/a
27.286A 27.293 27.287	Any amount not for personal use	0–5 yrs. & $15,000	0–10 yrs. & $30,000	0–5 yrs. & $15,000	0–5 yrs. & $15,000
	More than 100 lbs. imported into state	0–25 yrs. & $50,000	0–50 yrs. & $100,000	n/a	0–25 yrs. & $50,000
Massachusetts 94C.1 94C.31	Any amount	Probation	0–6 mos. & $500	0–2 yrs. & $5000	1–2 yrs. & $5000
94C.34 94C.32C.	50–100 lbs.			Mandatory 1 yr. & $500–10,000	Mandatory 1 yr. & $500–10,000

State & Statute	Amount	Possession: 1st Offense	Possession: 2nd Offense	Cultivation	Sale
Massachusetts (cont.)	100–2000 lbs.			Mandatory 3 yrs. & $2500–25,000	Mandatory 3 yrs. & $2500–25,000
	2000–10,000 lbs.			Mandatory 5 yrs. & $5000–50,000	Mandatory 5 yrs. & $5000–50,000
	More than 10,000 lbs.			Mandatory 10 yrs. & $20,000–200,000	Mandatory 10 yrs. & $20,000–200,000
Michigan 333.7403	Any amount	0–1 yr. & $1000	0–2 yrs. & $2000	0–4 yrs. & $2000	0–4 yrs. & $2000
Minnesota 152.01 152.02 152.15	Up to 1½ oz.	$0–100	0–90 days & $500	0–5 yrs. & $15,000	0–5 yrs. & $15,000
	More than 1½ oz.	0–3 yrs. & $3000	0–6 yrs. & $5000	0–5 yrs. & $15,000	0–5 yrs. & $15,000
Mississippi 41.29.105 41.29.115	Up to 1 oz. (not in vehicle)	$100–250	5–60 days & $250	0–10 yrs. & $15,000	0–20 yrs. & $30,000
41.29.139 41.29.147	Up to 1 oz. (in vehicle)	0–90 days & $500	0–180 days & $1000	0–10 yrs. & $15,000	0–20 yrs. & $30,000
	1 oz.–1 kilo (2.2 lbs.)	0–3 yrs. & $3000	0–6 yrs. & $6000	0–10 yrs. & $15,000	0–20 yrs. & $30,000

State & Statute	Amount	Possession: 1st Offense	Possession: 2nd Offense	Cultivation	Sale
Mississippi (cont.)	More than 1 kilo	Mandatory 3 yrs. & $10,000	Mandatory 5 yrs. & $20,000	0–10 yrs. & $15,000	3–20 yrs. & $30,000
Missouri 195.010 195.017	Up to 35 grams	0–1 yr. & $1000	0–5 yrs. & $1000	0–5 yrs. & $1000	5 yrs.–life
195.200	Over 35 grams	0–5 yrs. & $1000	0–5 yrs. & $1000	0–5 yrs. & $1000	5 yrs.–life
Montana 45.9.101 through 45.9.103	Up to 60 grams	0–1 yr. & $1000	0–3 yrs. & $1000	1 yr.–life	1 yr.–life
	More than 60 grams	0–5 yrs.	0–5 yrs.	1 yr.–life	1 yr.–life
Nebraska 28.401	Up to 1 oz.	$100	0–5 days & $200	0–5 yrs. & $10,000	0–20 yrs. & $10,000
28.405 28.416	1 oz.–1 lb.	0–7 days & $500	0–7 days & $500	0–5 yrs. & $10,000	0–20 yrs. & $10,000
	More than 1 lb.	0–5 yrs. & $10,000	0–5 yrs. & $10,000	0–5 yrs. & $10,000	0–20 yrs. & $10,000
Nevada 453.096 453.161 453.337	Up to 1 oz. by a person under 21	0–6 yrs. & $1000	1–6 yrs. & $5000	1–15 yrs. & $5000	1–15 yrs. & $5000
453.336	Any amount, all other ages	0–6 yrs. & $5000	1–10 yrs. & $20,000	1–15 yrs. & $5000	1–15 yrs. & $5000
New Hampshire 318B.26	Up to 1 lb.	0–1 yr. & $1000	0–7 yrs. & $2000	0–15 yrs. & $2000	0–15 yrs. & $2000

State & Statute	Amount	Possession: 1st Offense	Possession: 2nd Offense	Cultivation	Sale
New Hampshire (cont.)	More than 1 lb.	0–7 yrs. & $2000	0–15 yrs. & $2000	0–15 yrs. & $2000	0–15 yrs. & $2000
New Jersey 24.21.5	Up to 25 grams	0–6 mos. & $500	0–6 mos. & $500	0–5 yrs. & $15,000	0–5 yrs. & $15,000
24.21.2 24.21.19 24.21.20	More than 25 grams	0–5 yrs. & $15,000	0–5 yrs. & $15,000	0–5 yrs. & $15,000	0–5 yrs. & $15,000
New Mexico 30.31.2	Up to 1 oz.	0–15 days & $50–100	0–1 yr. & $100–1000	9 yrs. & $0–10,000	18 mos. & $0–5000
30.31.6 30.31.22 30.31.23	1–8 oz.	0–1 yr. & $100–1000	0–1 yr. & $100–1000	9 yrs. & $0–10,000	18 mos. & $0–5000
30.31.28	8 oz.–100 lbs.	0–5 yrs. & $5000	1–5 yrs. & $5000	9 yrs. & $0–10,000	18 mos. & $0–5000
31.18.15	Over 100 lbs.	3 yrs. & $0–5000	9 yrs. & $0–10,000	9 yrs. & $0–10,000	18 mos. & $0–5000
New York Penal 221.00 through 221.55	Up to 25 grams in private	$0–100	$0–200	0–1 yr. & $1000	0–1 yr. & $1000
Public Health 3382	25 grams–2 oz., or 2 oz. in public	0–3 mos. & $500	0–3 mos. & $500	0–1 yr. & $1000	0–4 yrs.

State & Statute	Amount	Possession: 1st Offense	Possession: 2nd Offense	Cultivation	Sale
3306	2–4 oz.	0–1 yr. & $1000	0–1 yr. & $1000	0–1 yr. & $1000	0–4 yrs.
3302	4–8 oz.	0–1 yr. & $1000	0–1 yr. & $1000	0–1 yr. & $1000	0–7 yrs.
	8 oz.–1 lb.	0–4 yrs.	0–4 yrs.	0–4 yrs.	0–7 yrs.
	1–10 lbs.	0–7 yrs.	0–7 yrs.	0–7 yrs.	0–15 yrs.
	Over 10 lbs.	0–15 yrs.	0–15 yrs.	0–15 yrs.	0–15 yrs.
North Carolina 90.87	Up to 1 oz.	$100	$100	$100	0–5 yrs. & $5000
90.94	1 oz.–50 lbs.	0–5 yrs. & $5000	0–5 yrs. & $5000	0–5 yrs. & $5000	0–5 yrs. & $5000
90.95 90.95(h)	50–100 lbs.	0–5 yrs. & $5000+	0–5 yrs. & $5000+	0–5 yrs. & $5000+	0–5 yrs. & $5000+
	100–2000 lbs.	7+ yrs. & $25,000+	7+ yrs. & $25,000+	7+ yrs. & $25,000+	7+ yrs. & $25,000+
	2000–10,000 lbs.	14 yrs.+ & $50,000+	14 yrs.+ & $50,000+	14 yrs.+ & $50,000+	14 yrs.+ & $50,000+
	10,000 lbs. or more	35 yrs.+ & $200,000	35 yrs.+ & $200,000	35 yrs.+ & $200,000	35 yrs.+ & $200,000
North Dakota 19.03.1. 01	Up to ½ oz. not in vehicle	0–30 days & $500	0–60 days & $1000	0–10 yrs. & $10,000	0–10 yrs. & $10,000
05 23	½–1 oz., or up to 1 oz. in vehicle	0–1 yr. & $1000	0–2 yrs. & $2000	0–10 yrs. & $10,000	0–10 yrs. & $10,000

309

State & Statute	Amount	Possession: 1st Offense	Possession: 2nd Offense	Cultivation	Sale
North Dakota (cont.)	More than 1 oz.	0–5 yrs. & $5000	0–5 yrs. & $5000	0–10 yrs. & $10,000	0–10 yrs. & $10,000
Ohio 2925.01 2925.11	Up to 100 grams	$0–100	$0–100	6 mos.–5 yrs. & $2500	6 mos.–5 yrs. & $2500
	100–200 grams	0–30 days & $250	0–30 days & $250	6 mos.–5 yrs. & $2500	6 mos.–5 yrs. & $2500
	200–600 grams	6 mos.–5 yrs. & $2500	1–10 yrs. & $5000	1–10 yrs. & $5000	1–10 yrs. & $5000
	More than 600 grams	1–10 yrs. & $5000	2–15 yrs. & $7500	2–15 yrs. & $7500	2–15 yrs. & $7500
Oklahoma 63.2.101 63.2.201 63.2.401 63.2.402	Any amount	0–1 yr.	2–10 yrs.	2–10 yrs. & $5000	2–10 yrs. & $5000
Oregon 475.005 475.992	Up to 1 oz.	$0–100	$0–100	0–10 yrs. & $2500	0–10 yrs. & $2500
	More than 1 oz.	0–10 yrs. & $2500	0–10 yrs. & $2500	0–10 yrs. & $2500	0–10 yrs. & $2500
Pennsylvania 35.780.	Up to 30 grams	0–30 days & $500	0–30 days & $500	0–5 yrs. & $15,000	0–5 yrs. & $15,000

310

State & Statute	Amount	Possession: 1st Offense	Possession: 2nd Offense	Cultivation	Sale
113	More than 30 grams	0–1 yr. & $5000	0–3 yrs. & $25,000	0–3 yrs. & $25,000	0–3 yrs. & $25,000
Rhode Island 21.28. 1.02 2.08 4.01 4.11	Any amount	0–1 yr. & $500	0–2 yrs. & $1000	0–30 yrs. & $50,000	0–30 yrs. & $50,000
South Carolina 44.53 370 190 110	Up to 1 oz.	0–30 days & $100–200	0–1 yr. & $200–1000	0–5 yrs. & $5000	0–5 yrs. & $5000
	More than 1 oz.	0–6 mos. & $1000	0–1 yr. & $2000	0–5 yrs. & $5000	0–5 yrs. & $5000
	10–100 lbs. (presumed for sale)			1–10 yrs. & $10,000	1–10 yrs. & $10,000
	100–2000 lbs. (presumed for sale)			5–25 yrs. & $25,000	5–25 yrs. & $25,000
	2000–10,000 lbs. (presumed for sale)			10–25 yrs. & $50,000	10–25 yrs. & $50,000
	Over 10,000 lbs. (presumed for sale)			15–30 yrs. & $200,000	15–30 yrs. & $200,000
South Dakota 22.42.1	Up to 1 oz.	0–30 days & $100	0–30 days & $100	0–30 days & $100	0–1 yr. & $1000

State & Statute	Amount	Possession: 1st Offense	Possession: 2nd Offense	Cultivation	Sale
22.42.6 22.42.7	1–8 oz.	0–1 yr. & $1000	0–1 yr. & $1000	0–1 yr. & $1000	0–2 yrs. & $2000
	8 oz.–1 lb.	0–1 yr. & $1000	0–1 yr. & $1000	0–1 yr. & $1000	0–5 yrs. & $5000
	Over 1 lb.	0–2 yrs. & $2000	0–2 yrs. & $2000	0–2 yrs. & $2000	0–5 yrs. & $5000
Tennessee 52.1409 52.1422 52.1432	Up to ½ oz.	0–1 yr. & $1000	1–2 yrs.	1–5 yrs. & $3000	0–1 yr. & $1000
	More than ½ oz.	0–1 yr. & $1000	1–2 yrs.	1–5 yrs. & $3000	1–5 yrs. & $3000
Texas 4476.15 1.02 2.03 4.05 4.01	Up to 2 oz.	0–180 days & $1000	30–180 days & $1000	0–180 days & $1000	2–10 yrs. & $5000
	2–4 oz.	0–1 yr. & $2000	90 days–1 yr. & $2000	0–1 yr. & $2000	2–10 yrs. & $5000
	4 oz.–50 lbs.	2–10 yrs. & $5000	2–20 yrs. & $10,000	2–10 yrs. & $5000	2–10 yrs. & $5000
	Over 50 lbs.	Up to life & $500,000	Up to life & $500,000	Up to life & $500,000	Up to life & $500,000
Utah 58.37.2 58.37.4 58.37.8	Any amount	0–6 mos. & $299	0–1 yr. & $1000	0–5 yrs. & $5000	0–5 yrs. & $5000

State & Statute	Amount	Possession: 1st Offense	Possession: 2nd Offense	Cultivation	Sale
Vermont T.18 4201	Up to ½ oz.	0–6 mos. & $500	0–2 yrs. & $2000	0–5 yrs. & $5000	0–5 yrs. & $5000
4224	½–2 oz.	0–3 yrs. & $3000	0–3 yrs. & $3000	0–5 yrs. & $5000	0–5 yrs. & $5000
	More than 2 oz.	0–5 yrs. & $5000	0–5 yrs. & $5000	0–5 yrs. & $5000	0–5 yrs. & $5000
Virginia 18.2 247.1	Up to ½ oz.	0–30 days & $500	0–1 yr. & $1000	0–30 days & $500	0–1 yr. & $1000
248.1	½ oz.–2 lbs.	0–30 days & $500	0–1 yr. & $1000	0–30 days & $500	0–10 yrs. & $1000
	More than 2 oz.	0–30 days & $500	0–1 yr. & $1000	5–30 yrs.	5–30 yrs.
Washington 69.50 101	Up to 40 grams	0–90 days & $250	0–90 days & $250	0–5 yrs. & $10,000	0–5 yrs. & $10,000
204	More than 40 grams	0–5 yrs. & $10,000	0–10 yrs. & $10,000	0–5 yrs. & $10,000	0–5 yrs. & $10,000
West Virginia 1.101 2.204	Any amount	3–6 mos. & $1000	3 mos.–1 yr. & $2000	1–5 yrs. & $15,000	1–5 yrs. & $15,000
	(Possession of less than 15 grams: presumption is against intent to distribute. Can get conditional discharge.)				
Wisconsin 161.01 161.14 161.41	Any amount	0–30 days & $500	0–30 days & $500	0–15 yrs. & $15,000	0–5 yrs. & $15,000

State & Statute	Amount	Possession: 1st Offense	Possession: 2nd Offense	Cultivation	Sale
Wyoming 35.7 1002 1014 1031 1038 1040	Any amount	0–6 mos. & $1000	0–1 yr. & $2000	0–6 mos. & $1000	0–10 yrs. & $10,000
District of Columbia 33.401	Any amount	0–1 yr. & $100–1000	0–10 yrs. & $500–5000	0–1 yr. & $100–1000	0–1 yr. & $100–1000
Federal Law 21 USC.841	Any amount	0–1 yr. & $5000	0–2 yrs. & $10,000	0–5 yrs. & $15,000	0–5 yrs. & $15,000

Notes

INTRODUCTION

Knowles, J., Ed. *Doing Better and Feeling Worse: Health in the United States.* New York: W. W. Norton, 1977, page 80.

CHAPTER ONE

1. Adapted from the pamphlet entitled *Drinking Etiquette* printed by the National Institute on Alcoholism and Alcohol Abuse, 1980.
2. Body weight standards taken from *The Book of Health—A Complete Guide to Making Health Last a Lifetime.* E. L. Wynder (Ed.), Franklin Watts, New York, 1981, page 289.
3. Mayer, Jean. *A Diet for Living,* David McKay Company, New York, page 65.
4. Erikson, E. H. *Childhood and Society,* W. W. Norton & Company, New York, 1963, page 80.
5. Freud, S. *A General Introduction to Psychoanalysis,* Washington Square Press, Inc., New York, 1963, page 364.
6. Fuqua, P. *Drug Abuse: Investigation and Control,* Gregg Division, McGraw-Hill Book Company, New York, page 12.

CHAPTER TWO

1. Rachal, V. J. et al. *Adolescent Drinking Behavior, Volume I, The Extent and Nature of Adolescent Alcohol and Drug Use: The 1974 and 1978 National Sample Studies,*

315

Center for the Study of Social Behavior, Research Triangle Institute, October 1980, adapted from page 52.

2. Farley, E. C., Santo, Y. and Speck, D. W. Multiple Drug Abuse Patterns of Youths in Treatment. Chapter in *Youth Drug Abuse: Problems, Issues, and Treatment,* Beschner, G. M. and Friedman, A. S. (Eds.) Lexington Books, Lexington, Mass., 1979, page 154.

3. Ingalls, Z. Higher Education's Drinking Problem, *The Chronicle of Higher Education,* Volume XXIV, Number 21, July 21, 1982, page 1.

4. Daum, M. and Lavenhar, M. A. *Religiosity and Drug Use: A Study of Jewish and Gentile College Students,* Services Research Report, National Institute on Drug Abuse, U.S. Department of Health, Education and Welfare, 1980, page 20.

5. *New York Times,* Life and Death of a Campus Drug Dealer, Sunday, September 5, 1982, page 1.

CHAPTER THREE

1. National Clearinghouse for Alcohol Information, National Institute on Alcohol Abuse and Alcoholism, *Alcohol and the Military,* Alcohol Topics In Brief, RPO 362, February 1982, page 2.

2. Levy, S. J. A Study of Drug Related Crime in Business and Industry. Chapter in *Drug Abuse in Industry: Growing Corporate Dilemma,* Scher, J. M. (Ed.), Charles C. Thomas, Springfield, Ill., 1973, pages 143–157.

3. Slaby, A. E. et al. *Handbook of Psychiatric Emergencies: A Guide for Emergencies in Psychiatry,* Medical Examination Publishing Company, Flushing, New York, 1975, page 70.

4. Selye, H. *Stress Without Distress,* Signet, 1974.

5. Reese, D. and Underwood, J. I'm Not Worth a Damn, *Sports Illustrated,* Volume 56, No. 24, June 14, 1982, page 1.

6. List adapted from *New York Times* article entitled New Health Plans focus on "Wellness," August 24, 1981, page D7.

CHAPTER FOUR

1. Preston, T. *The Clay Pedestal: A Re-examination of the Doctor Patient Relationship,* Madrona Publishers, Seattle, 1981, back flap.

2. Smith, M. C. and Knapp, D. *Pharmacy, Drugs and Medical Care,* Williams and Wilkins Company, Baltimore, 1972, pages 173 and 174.

3. Task Force on Women, *Deciding About Drugs—A Woman's Choice,* National Institute on Drug Abuse, U.S. Department of Health, Education and Welfare, 1979, page 13.

4. Burack, R. *The New Handbook of Prescription Drugs,* Ballantine, New York, 1976, p. xxii.

5. Medical News. Physician Prescribing Practices Criticized; Solutions in Question. *Journal of the American Medical Association,* 241:2353–2360, 1979.

6. Table adapted from Prescription Drug Abuse, *Consumers' Research Magazine,* January 1983, Volume 65, No. 1, page 25.

7. Hastings, A. C., Fadiman, J. and Gordon, J. S. *Health for the Whole Person—The Complete Guide to Holistic Medicine,* Bantam Books, New York, 1981, pages 17–26.

CHAPTER FIVE

1. Mack, R. E. What's Really in Alcoholic Drinks?, *Update: News about Alcoholism and Related Issues*, New York City Affiliate, Inc., National Council on Alcoholism, Vol. III, No. 7, November–December 1982, page 5.
2. Morgan, J. P., and Kagan, D. Street Amphetamine Quality and the Controlled Substance Act of 1970, *Journal of Psychoactive Drugs*, Vol. 10(4), 1978.
3. Jones, E. *The Life and Work of Sigmund Freud*, Anchor Doubleday, Garden City, New York, 1963, page 55.
4. Table adapted from Bush, P. J. *Drugs, Alcohol and Sex*, Marek, New York, 1980, pages 255–258 and Long, J. W. *The Essential Guide to Prescription Drugs*, Harper and Row, New York, 1980, page 809.

Index

321

Amphetamines, 271–272
  with alcohol, 240–241
  dealer substitutions for, 221, 222
  deaths and emergencies from, 205
  and pregnancy, 165
  in schools, 64t, 65t, 68t
  side effects of, 271–272
  in sports, 143
  uses for, 220, 222
  for women, 196
Amyl nitrates, 60t, 286–287
Anacin, 190–191
Analgesic drugs, 207
  advertising claims for, 190–191
  (*See also Specific types*)
Angel dust (*see* PCP)
Anslinger, Harry, 15
Antibiotics, tetracycline in, 178
Antidepressants, 283–284
  with alcohol, 241
  side effects of, 283–284
  tricyclic, 284
Antihistamines:
  activity limitations with, 171
  with alcohol, 241
Antipsychotic drugs, 280–281
Aphrodisiacs:
  drugs as, 242–252
    cocaine, 228
    methaqualone, 232, 233
    placebo effect in, 244
  Spanish Fly, 244–245
Army, U.S., drug use in, 108–110
Aspirin, 175, 193
  drug interactions with, 173
  in pain relief products, 190, 191
  in pregnancy, 164
Athletes, drug use by, 84–85, 140–143
Autogenic training, 213–214
Automobile accidents, alcohol-related, 32–33, 67, 69, 257–261
  (*See also* Drunk driving)

Bachman, Jerald, 59
Barbiturates, 278–279
  with alcohol, 240, 279
  in pregnancy, 165

  in schools, 60t, 64t, 65, 68t
  side effects of, 278
Belushi, John, 227
Bhang, 285
Biofeedback, 213
Bladder cancer, caffeine and, 120
Blood alcohol content (BAC), body weight and, 257
Bootlegs, 222
Brain function, nutrients and, 138
Breast feeding, drug use in, 164, 272, 281
Brompton's Mixture, 208
Bufferin, 190
Burack, Richard, 189
Butyl nitrates, 60t, 286–287

Caffeine:
  with cigarette smoking, 120
  daily consumption of, 115, 118
  in food and drugs, 116–117, 273–274
  health effects of, 118–121, 274
  hyperactivity and, 138
  intake reduction for, 121–123
  intoxification, 75–76, 114–115
  in pregnancy, 120–121
  (*See also* Coffee drinking)
Cancer:
  and cigarette smoking, 125, 126, 129
    passive inhalation in, 54
  coffee drinking and, 120
  marijuana smoking in, 47
Cannabis (*see* Marijuana)
Carbohydrates, craving for, 138
Cardiopulmonary resuscitation (CPR), 262–270
"Chasing the dragon," 234
Childproof container caps, 166
Children:
  accidental poisoning of, 166–167
  alcohol consumption by, 59, 60t, 61t, 62, 64t, 66–67, 68–69, 72–74
  choking first aid for, 267
  of drug abusers, 50–54
  drug free modeling by, 99–103
  drug use by:
    clique membership and, 82–84
    family influence on, 1–4

INDEX

Medications (*cont.*)
  in homeopathic medicine, 215
  me-too products, 189–190
  patient knowledge of, 156–158
  pharmacist advice on, 184, 185–186
  phenacetin in, 209–210
  physician knowledge of, 188–189, 191–
    192
  sexual function and, 245, 246–247
  side effects of, 161–162
  storage and dating of, 166–167
  withdrawal effects of, 174
  (*See also* Over-the counter (OTC) drugs;
    Prescription drugs)
Medicine (*see* Holistic medicine)
Meditation, 214
Memory, stimulant drugs and, 74–75
Meprobamate (Dalmane), 280
Mescaline, 285, 286
Methaqualone, 279
  adulterated, 232
  alcohol consumption with, 233
  as aphrodisiac, 232, 233
  dealer substitutions for, 221, 222
  deaths and emergencies from, 204
  prescription of, 231–232
  in schools, 60t
  side effects of, 233, 279
Methylxanthines, 118
Miller, Sanford, 119, 120
Monoamine oxidase (*see* MAO)
Morgan, John, 222
Morphine, 207, 208, 240
Mothers Against Drunk Drivers (MADD),
  259, 260
Murphy, Samuel, Jr., 191

Nasal septum, perforation of, 229
Nasal spray, dependency upon, 209
National Council on Alcoholism (NCA),
  296
National Football League (NFL), cocaine
  use in, 140–141
National Organization for the Reform of
  Marijuana Laws (NORML), 18
National Organization for Women (NOW),
  201
Neurotransmitters, 138

New Handbook of Prescription Drugs, The
  (Burack), 189
New York Telephone Company, 145
Nicotine, 124–125, 273
  (*See also* Cigarette smoking)
Nonprescription drugs (*see* Over-the
  counter drugs)
Norepinephrine, 138

Obesity:
  body fat and, 5
  family influence on, 2, 4–5, 6–7
  fat cell hypothesis of, 6
  health risks of, 133
  incidence of, 6
  (*See also* Eating behavior)
Objective confrontation process, 43–44
O'Malley, Patrick, 59
Opiates, 282–283
  in over-the-counter (OTC) drugs, 206–
    207
  in schools, 60t, 61t, 68t
  (*See also Specific types*)
Oral contraceptives, contraindications to,
  168–169
Orgasm, 248, 249
Orinase, 158
Ornade, 158
Over-the-counter (OTC) drugs, 68t
  addictive, 206–207, 209–210
  advertising claims for, 190–191
  antihistamines in, 171
  caffeine content of, 117
  for children, 178
  cocaine in, 225
  in pregnancy, 165–166
    aspirin, 164
  (*See also* Cold remedies; Medications)
Overweight (*see* Obesity)

Pain management:
  drug use for, 8–12
    by athletes, 141–142
    by hospice movement, 208
    of over-the counter (OTC) drugs, 206–
      208
  family model for, 12–13
  self honesty in, 11–12

327

INDEX

Religion, and drug use, 69–70
Rockers (clique), 83

St. Christopher's hospice, London, 208
Salt:
  elimination of, 137
  health problems from, 136
Sativa, 237
Schools and colleges:
  alcohol consumption in, 59, 60t, 61t, 62,
    64t, 66–69, 72
  drug use in, 58
    availability and, 64–65
    clique membership and, 82–83
    grade of first use, 59, 60t
    of LSD, 70–71
    of multiple substances, 67–68
    parental action in, 73–74
    peer influence on, 62, 63t, 64, 78–82
    prevalence and recency of, 59, 61–62
    prevention programs for, 87–94
    religiosity and, 69–70
    risk factors for, 69–70, 72
    sports and, 84–85
    as study aids, 74–78
Sedatives:
  alcohol consumption with, 240, 274–277
  barbiturates, 278–279
  contraindications for, 277
  nonbarbiturates, 279
  in schools, 60t, 61t, 64t
  side effects of, 277–278
  (*See also* Tranquilizers)
Seizures, warning signs of, 264, 268
Selye, Hans, 129, 130
Serotonin, 138
Sexual function:
  and drug enhancers, 242–252
    cocaine, 228
    methaqualone, 232, 233
  drug interference with, 245, 246–247,
    249, 283
  medication effects on, 171
Sexual response cycle, drug effects on, 248
Side effects, 271–287
  in drug therapy, 161–162
  pharmacist advice on, 185–186
  from pleasure drugs, 219–220

Sinsemilla, 236–237
Smoking (*see* Cigarette smoking;
    Marijuana)
Smuts, Jan Christiaan, 150
Soda, caffeine content of, 116–117
Sopor (*see* Methaqualone)
Spanish Fly, 244–245
Speed (*see* Amphetamines)
Speedball, 227
Sports, and drug use, 84–85, 140–143
Spyker, Daniel, 167
Stepping stone theory, of drug use, 71–72
Steroids, 141–142
Stimulant drugs, 271–274
  alcohol consumption with, 240–241
  caffeine in, 117
  effects on memory, 74–75
  in schools, 60t, 61t
  as study aids, 74–75
  in sports, 143
  (*See also Specific types*)
STP (2, 5-dimethoxy-4-methyl-
    amphetamine), 261–262, 285, 286
Street drugs (*see* Pleasure drugs)
Stress:
  defined, 129–130
  eating behavior and, 131
  smoking and, 130–131
Stroke, warning signs of, 264
Sugar:
  effect on mood, 138, 139
  elimination of, 137
  health problems from, 136
Sulfur dioxide, in alcoholic beverages,
    218
Supra-additive, 239
Synergism, 239

Talwin (*see* Pentazocine)
Tardive dyskinesia, 281
Tea, caffeine content of, 116
Tetracycline:
  in medications, 178
  side effects of, 177
Tetrahydrocannabinol (*see* THC)
THC (tetrahydrocannabinol), 8–9, 39
  in marijuana, 236, 237, 240, 285
Theophylline, 273

About the Author

Stephen J. Levy, Ph.D., a psychologist specializing in the treatment of alcohol and other drug abuse, is former director of both the Division of Drug Abuse at the New Jersey Medical School and the Alcohol Treatment Program at Beth Israel Medical Center. Dr. Levy is currently Adjunct Associate Professor of Psychology at John Jay College of Criminal Justice, City University of New York, and acts as private consultant to corporate employee assistance programs. He has served on the faculties of Hunter College, Empire State College, New Jersey Medical School, and the Mount Sinai School of Medicine. He maintains a private practice in psychotherapy in New York City and Nanuet, New York, where he lives with his family.

Catalog

If you are interested in a list of fine Paperback
books, covering a wide range of subjects
and interests, send your name and address,
requesting your free catalog, to:

McGraw-Hill Paperbacks
1221 Avenue of Americas
New York, N. Y. 10020